LUPUS COOKBOOK

The Ultimate Easy-to-Follow Recipes for Living with Lupus

EVELYN LATTORE

TABLE OF CONTENTS

INTRODUCTION

A balanced and nutritious diet is essential for managing symptoms of autoimmune disorders, such as lupus, by helping to control inflammation linked to gut health issues.

The gastrointestinal tract, home to the majority of the immune system and known as the microbiome, plays a crucial role in overall health.

Up to 90% of all diseases can be traced back to gut dysfunction, highlighting the importance of a targeted lupus diet for effective treatment.

According to the Lupus Foundation of America, a lack of specific diet and nutrition information for lupus patients remains a significant challenge. However, research has revealed how certain foods and lifestyle choices can mitigate the adverse effects of lupus by influencing the body's inflammatory response.

A diet tailored to support lupus patients can enhance gut health by addressing allergies, deficiencies, and oxidative stress.

Given the overlap between lupus symptoms and other autoimmune conditions, a diet low in processed foods and rich in antioxidants is crucial for managing various related symptoms.

Key nutrients such as fiber and antioxidants are most beneficial when sourced from whole foods rather than supplements. A lupus-friendly diet emphasizes healthy fats, abundant vegetables and fruits, and probiotic-rich foods.

This approach can also offer broader protective benefits, as individuals with lupus face an increased risk of chronic health issues, such as heart disease, compared to the general population.

Lupus is a chronic autoimmune disorder where the immune system mistakenly attacks healthy tissues and organs. This can lead to inflammation and damage across various body systems, including the heart, joints, brain, kidneys, lungs, and endocrine glands such as the adrenals and thyroid.

The exact cause of lupus is not fully understood, but several risk factors have been identified:

- **Genetics:** Individuals with a family history of lupus or other autoimmune disorders may have an increased risk.
- **Gender:** Women make up 90% of lupus cases.
- **Age:** Women aged 15 to 45 are most likely to develop lupus.
- **Ethnicity:** African-American, Asian, and Native American women experience lupus two to three times more often than Caucasians.
- **Diet and Nutrition:** Poor dietary habits and nutrient deficiencies may contribute to lupus risk.
- **Leaky Gut Syndrome:** This condition can exacerbate lupus symptoms.
- **Food Allergies and Sensitivities:** These can play a role in triggering lupus flare-ups.
- **Toxicity Exposure:** Contact with environmental toxins may increase the risk of developing lupus.

Lupus symptoms often include fatigue, headaches, joint discomfort, sleep disturbances, digestive issues, and skin rashes. Managing lupus can be challenging due to its complex diagnosis and treatment, and patients may also experience emotional effects such as anxiety, depression, memory problems, and insomnia related to the stress of the condition.

Standard lupus treatment typically consists of medications to control symptoms and lifestyle adjustments, including dietary improvements and exercise.

Patients may be prescribed multiple daily medications such as corticosteroids, NSAIDs, thyroid medications, and hormone replacement therapies.

Despite these medications, following an anti-inflammatory diet is crucial for addressing the underlying causes of lupus and alleviating symptoms.

IMPORTANCE OF DIETARY CHANGES

While no specific diet can universally treat lupus, adopting a healthy lupus diet can help prevent flare-ups and minimize complications.

Inflammation associated with lupus and other autoimmune reactions stems from an overactive immune response and compromised gut health. Leaky gut syndrome may develop in lupus patients, causing the gut lining to allow particles into the bloodstream, triggering an autoimmune response.

This inflammatory process can increase the risk of various health issues, such as heart disease, hypertension, weight gain, joint damage, and bone loss. The microbiome, a complex community of trillions of bacteria, plays a key role in inflammation and overall health.

It influences nutrient absorption, hormone production, and protection against environmental toxins. These bacterial populations fluctuate based on diet, sleep quality, daily exposure to bacteria or chemicals, and emotional stress levels.

Our diet plays a significant role in shaping our microbiota, as the foods we consume can either cause oxidative stress, allergies, and deficiencies or improve our immunity, hormonal balance, and overall health.

Eating whole foods high in probiotics, antioxidants, and prebiotic fiber can lower inflammation by promoting beneficial gut bacteria. These foods also fight free radical damage, offering anti-aging benefits to those without lupus or other immune disorders.

TOP LUPUS DIET FOODS

- **Organic, Unprocessed Foods:** Eating foods in their natural, whole form helps minimize exposure to synthetic additives, toxins, and pesticides often found in packaged and non-organic foods. For lupus patients with compromised immune systems, avoiding synthetic chemicals and heavy metals is crucial for recovery.

- **Raw and Cooked Vegetables:** Consuming vegetables in both raw and cooked forms supports an alkaline body environment and lowers inflammation. Vegetables provide antioxidants, prebiotics, fiber, and essential vitamins and minerals. Some of the best choices include leafy greens, garlic, onions, asparagus, artichokes, bell peppers, beets, mushrooms, and avocados. Aim for variety and at least four to five servings per day.
- **Fresh Fruit:** Fresh fruit offers vital nutrients like vitamins C and E, which can be challenging to obtain from other sources. Berries, pomegranates, and cherries are particularly beneficial due to their high antioxidant content.
- **Wild-Caught Fish:** Wild seafood provides omega-3 fats, which reduce inflammation. Options such as wild salmon, sardines, mackerel, halibut, trout, and anchovies are excellent choices. Consume these fish two to three times per week or consider supplements if needed. Opt for "wild-caught" fish to avoid heavy metals and other contaminants found in farm-raised varieties.
- **Probiotic Foods:** Probiotic-rich foods, including yogurt, kefir, kombucha, and cultured vegetables such as sauerkraut and kimchi, support gut health by introducing beneficial bacteria.
- **Bone Broth:** Bone broth, rich in collagen, glutathione, and trace minerals, can alleviate autoimmune and inflammatory symptoms linked to lupus. Aim to consume eight to sixteen ounces of bone broth daily, either as a beverage or in soups.
- **Herbs, Spices, and Teas:** Incorporating herbs and spices such as turmeric, ginger, basil, oregano, thyme, and green tea into your diet can provide additional health benefits.
- **Hydration:** Drinking water, herbal tea, and green tea supports skin health and overall hydration.

WORST INFLAMMATORY FOODS TO AVOID ON THE LUPUS DIET

- **Trans and Hydrogenated Fats:** Found in packaged and fried foods, these fats should be avoided. Opt for home cooking and limit fast food, processed meats, and sweets.
- **Refined Vegetable Oils:** Cheap oils such as canola, corn, safflower, sunflower, and soybean are high in pro-inflammatory omega-6 fatty acids and should be minimized.
- **Pasteurized Dairy Products:** Conventional dairy often contains allergens due to homogenization and pasteurization, which strip important enzymes.
- **Refined Carbohydrates and Processed Grains:** Low in nutrients and often containing gluten, these foods can hinder digestion and contribute to inflammation.
- **Conventional Meat, Poultry, and Eggs:** Farm-raised products can be higher in omega-6 fats, which may negatively impact the consumer's microbiome. Choose high-quality, organic, or pasture-raised options.
- **Added Sugars:** Excess sugar can cause blood sugar fluctuations, mood swings, and inflammation. Avoid packaged snacks, breads, condiments, dairy, canned goods, and cereals with added sugars.
- **High-Sodium Foods:** Lupus can affect the kidneys, so it's essential to limit sodium intake to avoid fluid retention, swelling, and electrolyte imbalances. High-sodium foods include condiments, processed meats, canned soups, frozen meals, and fried foods.
- **Alcohol:** Excessive alcohol and caffeine consumption can exacerbate anxiety, worsen inflammation, impair liver function, increase pain, and lead to dehydration and sleep issues.
- **Caution with Certain Legumes:** Some legumes, such as alfalfa seeds and sprouts, green beans, peanuts, soybeans, and snow peas, contain a substance that may trigger lupus flare-ups in certain individuals. These reactions can result in symptoms such as antinuclear antibodies in the blood, muscle pains, fatigue, abnormal immune function, and kidney issues, potentially linked to the amino acid L-canavanine.

STRATEGIES TO MANAGE LUPUS SYMPTOMS

- **Smaller, More Frequent Meals:** If you experience indigestion, try eating four to six smaller meals throughout the day instead of three larger ones.
- **Moderate Fat Intake:** Since fat can be challenging to digest for those with lupus, opt for smaller portions of healthy fats and avoid high-fat meals. Healthy fats are essential for cognitive and hormonal health.
- **Vitamin D Supplementation:** Vitamin D plays a crucial role in immune system health and may impact bone metabolism, cognitive function, and hormone production. Low levels of vitamin D have been associated with an increased risk of autoimmune conditions and chronic diseases. Consult your doctor about supplementation, especially if you spend limited time outdoors.
- **Avoid Smoking and Recreational Drug Use:** Smoking and drug use can exacerbate lung damage and lead to complications, so it's best to avoid these substances.
- **Staying physically active is crucial for those with lupus:** Gentle exercises such as brisk walking, swimming, water aerobics, tai chi, yoga, cycling, Pilates, or using an elliptical machine for 20-30 minutes a day can improve overall health without exacerbating symptoms.
- **Manage Stress Levels:** Keeping emotional stress in check is vital for lupus management. Stressful situations and trauma can trigger flare-ups, increasing inflammation throughout the body. Utilize natural stress-relief methods to regulate cortisol levels and prevent triggering symptoms.
- **Prioritize Sleep and Rest:** Ensure you get seven to nine hours of quality sleep each night to promote healing and overall well-being. Additionally, take breaks during the day to relax and recharge.

To manage lupus effectively, prioritize a well-balanced diet rich in whole, unprocessed foods, including vegetables, fruits, clean proteins, probiotics, fiber, and antioxidants.

Avoid foods that can exacerbate inflammation, such as added sugars, refined vegetable oils, gluten-containing carbs, farm-raised animal products, and synthetic additives in packaged foods.

Additionally, some individuals benefit from limiting certain legumes, such as alfalfa, soybeans, and peanuts.

By reducing processed foods and focusing on fresh or raw options, as well as moderate amounts of healthy fats, grass-fed meats, and wild-caught fish, those with lupus can help prevent complications like heart disease, joint pain, and cognitive or mood issues.

This cookbook is designed specifically for individuals living with lupus, offering a variety of nourishing and delicious recipes that support overall health and help manage symptoms.

The recipes focus on whole, unprocessed foods rich in anti-inflammatory nutrients, antioxidants, and healthy fats that can promote gut health, support immune function, and reduce flare-ups.

By incorporating a diverse range of fruits, vegetables, lean proteins, healthy fats, and probiotics, you can create meals that are both satisfying and beneficial for your well-being.

The cookbook emphasizes foods that nourish the body, such as omega-3-rich fish, leafy greens, and colorful vegetables, while avoiding potential triggers like refined sugars, processed foods, and certain legumes.

Whether you're newly diagnosed or have been living with lupus for years, this guide provides valuable insights and resources to help you take control of your health and improve your quality of life.

Enjoy exploring these recipes and discovering new ways to support your body while savoring each delicious meal.

Breakfast Recipes

BANANA BREAD OATMEAL

🥣 **Preparation Time : 5 min**

🍴 **Cooking Time : 10 min**

🕐 **Servings : 1**

Ingredients

- 1/2 cup gluten-free oats
- 1 ripe banana, mashed
- 1 cup almond milk (unsweetened)
- 1/2 teaspoon ground cinnamon
- 1 tablespoon chia seeds
- 1 tablespoon walnuts, chopped (optional)
- 1 tablespoon maple syrup or honey (optional)
- Fresh banana slices for topping

Preparation

1. In a small saucepan, combine oats, almond milk, and mashed banana. Bring to a simmer over medium heat.
2. Cook for about 5-7 minutes, stirring occasionally, until the oats are tender and the mixture thickens.
3. Stir in the ground cinnamon and chia seeds.
4. If desired, add a drizzle of maple syrup or honey for sweetness.
5. Serve in a bowl and top with fresh banana slices and chopped walnuts.

Nutrition Value (Per Serving)

Calories: 250 - Protein: 6g - Fat: 9g - Carbohydrates: 37g - Fiber: 7g

OAT WAFFLES

Preparation Time : 10 min

Cooking Time : 10 min

Servings : 2

Ingredients

- 1 cup gluten-free oat flour
- 1/2 teaspoon baking powder
- 1/4 teaspoon ground cinnamon
- 1/2 cup unsweetened almond milk
- 1 egg or egg substitute
- 1 tablespoon coconut oil, melted
- 1 tablespoon honey or maple syrup
- 1/2 teaspoon vanilla extract
- Fresh berries and honey for topping (optional)

Preparation

1. In a mixing bowl, whisk together oat flour, baking powder, and ground cinnamon.
2. In a separate bowl, whisk together almond milk, egg, melted coconut oil, honey or maple syrup, and vanilla extract.
3. Combine the wet ingredients with the dry ingredients and mix until smooth.
4. Preheat your waffle iron and lightly grease with cooking spray or coconut oil.
5. Transfer half of the batter into the waffle iron and cook for the recommended amount of time (typically five minutes), as directed by the manufacturer.
6. Repeat with the remaining batter to make another waffle.
7. Serve the waffles warm with your choice of fresh berries and a drizzle of honey for added sweetness.

Nutrition Value (Per Serving)

Calories: 200- Protein: 6g - Fat: 9g - Carbohydrates: 25g- Fiber: 3g

CINNAMON APPLE PARFAIT

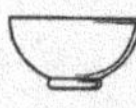 **Preparation Time : 10 min**

 **Cooking Time : 10 min**

 **Servings : 2**

Ingredients

- 2 peeled, cored, and sliced medium apples
- 1 tablespoon coconut oil
- 1 teaspoon ground cinnamon
- 1/4 cup chopped walnuts
- 1 cup dairy-free yogurt (such as coconut or almond yogurt)
- 1/4 cup gluten-free granola
- Maple syrup or honey (optional, for drizzling)

Preparation

1. In a skillet over medium heat, warm the coconut oil. Add diced apples and cook for 5-7 minutes, or until softened.
2. Sprinkle ground cinnamon over the apples and stir to coat evenly. Cook for another 2-3 minutes.
3. Remove from heat and let the cinnamon apples cool slightly.
4. In serving glasses or bowls, layer the cinnamon apples, chopped walnuts, dairy-free yogurt, and gluten-free granola.
5. Continue layering until all ingredients have been utilized, and then top with a granola layer.
6. Drizzle with maple syrup or honey if desired.
7. Serve immediately and enjoy!

Nutrition Value (Per Serving)

Calories: 320 kcal - Carbohydrates: 36g - Protein: 6g - Fat: 18g - Fiber: 6g - Sugar: 20g - Sodium: 60mg

BREAKFAST TOSTADAS

Preparation Time : 15 min

Cooking Time : 15 min

Servings : 2

Ingredients

- 4 gluten-free corn tortillas
- 1 cup cooked black beans
- 1 avocado, sliced
- 1 tomato, diced
- 1/4 cup chopped cilantro
- 1 lime, cut into wedges
- Salt and pepper, to taste
- Dairy-free yogurt or salsa (optional, for topping)

Preparation

1. Preheat the oven to 375°F (190°C).
2. Place corn tortillas on a baking sheet and bake for 10-12 minutes, or until crispy.
3. While the tortillas are baking, heat the black beans in a small saucepan over medium heat until warmed through.
4. Once the tortillas are crispy, remove them from the oven and assemble the tostadas.
5. Spread a layer of black beans on each tortilla, followed by sliced avocado, diced tomato, and chopped cilantro.
6. Squeeze fresh lime juice over the tostadas and season with salt and pepper to taste.
7. Serve immediately with dairy-free yogurt or salsa on the side, if desired.

Nutrition Value (Per Serving)

Calories: 280 kcal - Carbohydrates: 38g - Protein: 8g - Fat: 12g- Fiber: 12g - Sugar: 3g - Sodium: 230mg

MEDITERRANEAN BAKED SWEET POTATOES

🥣 **Preparation Time : 10 min**

✕ **Cooking Time : 45 min**

🕐 **Servings : 4**

Ingredients

- 4 medium sweet potatoes
- 1 tablespoon olive oil
- 1 teaspoon dried oregano
- 1 teaspoon dried basil
- 1/2 teaspoon garlic powder
- 1/2 teaspoon paprika
- Salt and pepper, to taste
- 1 cup cherry tomatoes, halved
- 1/2 cup sliced black olives
- 1/4 cup chopped fresh parsley
- Dairy-free yogurt or tahini sauce (optional, for serving)

Preparation

1. Preheat the oven to 400°F (200°C).
2. Scrub the sweet potatoes clean and pierce each one several times with a fork.
3. Place the sweet potatoes on a baking sheet lined with parchment paper and bake for 40-45 minutes, or until tender.
4. In a small bowl, whisk together olive oil, dried oregano, dried basil, garlic powder, paprika, salt, and pepper.
5. Remove the sweet potatoes from the oven and let them cool slightly.
6. Cut each sweet potato in half lengthwise and fluff the flesh with a fork.
7. Drizzle the olive oil mixture over the sweet potatoes, then top with cherry tomatoes, black olives, and chopped parsley.
8. Serve hot with dairy-free yogurt or tahini sauce on the side, if desired.

Nutrition Value (Per Serving)

Calories: 240 kcal - Carbohydrates: 45g - Protein: 4g - Fat: 5g - Fiber: 8g - Sugar: 9g - Sodium: 380mg

QUINOA BREAKFAST BOWL WITH FRESH BERRIES

🥣 **Preparation Time : 5 min**

🍴 **Cooking Time : 15 min**

🕐 **Servings : 2**

Ingredients

- 1 cup quinoa, rinsed
- 2 cups almond milk
- 1 tablespoon maple syrup
- 1 teaspoon ground cinnamon
- 1 cup of raw berries, like raspberries, blueberries, or strawberries
- 1/4 cup finely chopped nuts (almonds, pecans, or walnuts)
- Fresh mint leaves, for garnish (optional)

Preparation

1. In a saucepan, combine quinoa and almond milk.
2. Bring to a boil, then decrease heat to low, cover, and cook for 12-15 minutes, or until quinoa is tender and liquid has been absorbed.
3. Remove from heat and stir in maple syrup and ground cinnamon.
4. Divide the cooked quinoa into bowls.
5. Top each bowl with fresh berries and chopped nuts.
6. Garnish with fresh mint leaves if desired.
7. Serve warm and enjoy!

Nutrition Value (Per Serving)

Calories: 350 kcal - Carbohydrates: 55g - Protein: 10g - Fat: 10g - Fiber: 8g - Sugar: 12g - Sodium: 110mg

SPINACH AND MUSHROOM OMELETTE WITH AVOCADO SLICES

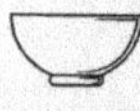 **Preparation Time : 10 min**

 **Cooking Time : 10 min**

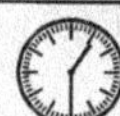 **Servings : 2**

Ingredients

- 4 large eggs
- 1 cup fresh spinach leaves
- 1/2 cup sliced mushrooms
- 1/4 cup diced onion
- 1 tablespoon olive oil
- 1 avocado, sliced
- Optional garnish: fresh herbs (e.g., parsley or chives)

Preparation

1. In a bowl, whisk together the eggs until well beaten. Set aside.
2. Heat the olive oil in a pan over medium heat. Add diced onion and sliced mushrooms, and cook until softened, about 3-4 minutes.
3. Add fresh spinach leaves to the skillet and cook until wilted, about 1-2 minutes.
4. Pour the beaten eggs onto the vegetables in the skillet. Cook until the edges start to set, then gently lift the edges with a spatula to let the uncooked eggs flow underneath.
5. Once the omelette is mostly set, fold it in half and cook for another minute to ensure the eggs are cooked through.
6. Carefully slide the omelette onto a plate and cut it in half.
7. Serve with avocado slices on the side.
8. Garnish with fresh herbs if desired.
9. Serve hot and enjoy!

Nutrition Value (Per Serving)

Calories: 320 kcal - Carbohydrates: 12g - Protein: 14g - Fat: 24g - Fiber: 7g - Sugar: 2g- Sodium: 120mg

OVERNIGHT CHIA SEED PUDDING

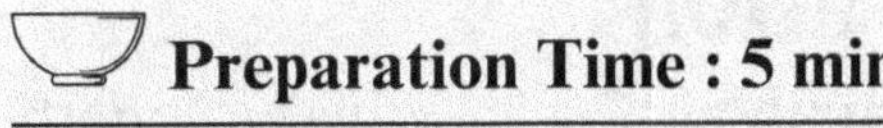

Preparation Time : 5 min

Cooking Time : 0 min

Servings : 2

Ingredients

- 1/4 cup chia seeds
- 1 cup almond milk
- 1 tablespoon maple syrup (optional)
- 1/2 teaspoon vanilla extract
- 1 ripe mango, diced
- Additional fresh berries, for garnish (optional)

Preparation

1. In a bowl or jar, combine chia seeds, almond milk, maple syrup (if using), and vanilla extract. Stir well to combine.
2. Cover and refrigerate overnight, or for at least 4 hours, until the chia pudding thickens.
3. Before serving, stir the chia pudding to redistribute the seeds evenly.
4. Divide the chia pudding into serving bowls or glasses.
5. Top with diced mango and additional fresh berries if desired.
6. Serve chilled and enjoy!

Nutrition Value (Per Serving)

Calories: 250 kcal - Carbohydrates: 34g - Protein: 7g - Fat: 10g - Fiber: 12g - Sugar: 20g- Sodium: 80mg

BUCKWHEAT PANCAKES WITH BLUEBERRY COMPOTE

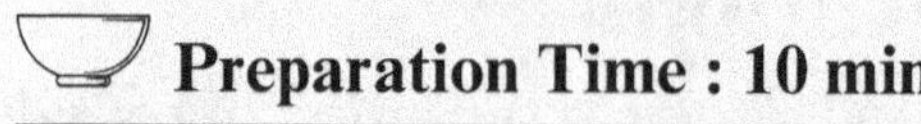

🥣 **Preparation Time : 10 min**

🍴 **Cooking Time : 15 min**

🕐 **Servings : 2**

Ingredients for Buckwheat Pancakes:

- 1 cup buckwheat flour
- 1 tablespoon baking powder
- 1 tablespoon maple syrup
- 1 cup almond milk
- 1 tablespoon coconut oil, melted
- Fresh blueberries for garnish (optional)

Ingredients for Blueberry Compote:

- 1 cup fresh or frozen blueberries
- 1 tablespoon maple syrup
- 1 tablespoon water
- 1 teaspoon lemon juice
- Lemon zest for garnish (optional)

Preparation

1. In a mixing bowl, whisk together buckwheat flour and baking powder.
2. Add maple syrup, almond milk, and melted coconut oil to the dry ingredients. Mix until well combined.
3. Heat a non-stick skillet over medium heat. Pour batter into the griddle to make pancakes of your desired size.
4. Cook pancakes for 2-3 minutes on each side, or until golden brown.
5. While pancakes are cooking, prepare the blueberry compote. In a small saucepan, combine blueberries, maple syrup, water, and lemon juice. Cook over low heat, stirring occasionally, until the blueberries burst and the mixture thickens slightly, about 5-7 minutes.
6. Serve pancakes topped with blueberry compote and garnish with fresh blueberries and lemon zest if desired.
7. Enjoy your delicious and nutritious breakfast!

Nutrition Value (Per Serving)

Calories: 350 kcal- Carbohydrates: 60g - Protein: 8g - Fat: 9g - Fiber: 10g- Sugar: 18g - Sodium: 30mg

EGG MUFFINS

<table>
<tr><td>

🥣 **Preparation Time : 10 min**

🍴 **Cooking Time : 20 min**

🕐 **Servings : 2**

Ingredients

- 4 large eggs
- 1 cup fresh spinach, chopped
- 1 tomato, diced
- 1/4 cup crumbled feta cheese
- Salt and pepper to taste
- Fresh herbs for garnish (optional)

</td><td>

Preparation

1. Preheat the oven to 350°F (175°C). Grease a muffin tin with olive oil or line with paper liners.
2. In a mixing bowl, whisk together eggs until well beaten. Season with salt and pepper.
3. Divide chopped spinach, diced tomato, and crumbled feta cheese evenly among the muffin cups.
4. Pour beaten eggs over the spinach, tomato, and feta in each muffin cup, filling them about 3/4 full.
5. Bake in the preheated oven for 15-20 minutes, or until the egg muffins are set and slightly golden on top.
6. Take out of the oven and allow it to cool down for several minutes before serving.
7. Garnish with fresh herbs if desired.
8. Enjoy these protein-packed egg muffins for a satisfying breakfast on the go!

</td></tr>
</table>

Nutrition Value (Per Serving)

Calories: 220 kcal - Carbohydrates: 6g - Protein: 15g - Fat: 15g - Fiber: 2g - Sugar: 3g - Sodium: 45mg

BREAKFAST BURRITO

<table>
<tr><td>

Preparation Time : 10 min

Cooking Time : 10 min

Servings : 2

</td></tr>
</table>

Ingredients

- 4 gluten-free tortillas
- 1 cup cooked black beans
- 1 cup fresh spinach
- 1 avocado, sliced
- Salsa or hot sauce for serving (optional)

Preparation

1. Heat the tortillas in a dry skillet over medium heat for about 30 seconds on each side, until warmed through.
2. In the same skillet, add cooked black beans and fresh spinach. Cook until spinach is wilted and beans are heated through, about 3-5 minutes.
3. Divide the black bean and spinach mixture evenly among the tortillas.
4. Top each tortilla with sliced avocado.
5. Roll up the tortillas to form burritos.
6. Serve immediately with salsa or hot sauce on the side if desired.
7. Enjoy these flavorful and nutritious breakfast burritos to start your day off right!

Nutrition Value (Per Serving)

Calories: 320 kcal - Carbohydrates: 38g - Protein: 10g - Fat: 14g
- Fiber: 12g - Sugar: 3g - Sodium: 40mg

ACAI BOWL

<table>
<tr><td>Preparation Time : 5 min</td></tr>
<tr><td>Cooking Time : 0 min</td></tr>
<tr><td>Servings : 1</td></tr>
</table>

Ingredients

- 1 packet frozen unsweetened acai puree
- 1/2 ripe banana, sliced
- 1/4 cup gluten-free granola
- 1 tablespoon coconut flakes
- Fresh berries for garnish (optional)

Preparation

1. Run the frozen acai puree packet under warm water for a few seconds to soften slightly.
2. Transfer the acai puree to a bowl.
3. Top with sliced banana, gluten-free granola, and coconut flakes.
4. Garnish with fresh berries if desired.
5. Serve immediately and enjoy this refreshing and nutritious acai bowl!

Nutrition Value (Per Serving)

Calories: 250 kcal - Carbohydrates: 35g - Protein: 2g - Fat: 12g - Fiber: 6g - Sugar: 15g - Sodium: 10mg

TURMERIC SCRAMBLED TOFU

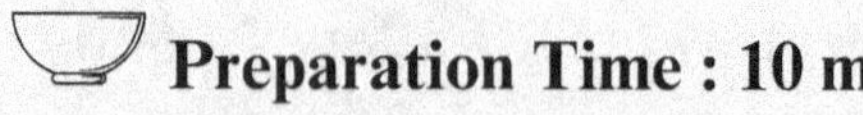

Preparation Time : 10 min

Cooking Time : 10 min

Servings : 2

Ingredients

- 1 block (about 14 oz) firm tofu, drained and crumbled
- 1 teaspoon ground turmeric
- 1/2 teaspoon ground cumin
- 1/2 teaspoon garlic powder
- Salt and pepper to taste
- 1 tablespoon olive oil
- 1 cup cherry tomatoes, halved
- 2 cups chopped kale

Preparation

1. In a bowl, combine crumbled tofu with ground turmeric, ground cumin, garlic powder, salt, and pepper. Mix well to coat the tofu evenly with spices.
2. In a skillet over medium heat, warm the olive oil. Add cherry tomatoes and cook for 2-3 minutes until slightly softened.
3. Add chopped kale to the skillet and cook for another 2-3 minutes until wilted.
4. Push the vegetables to one side of the skillet and add the seasoned tofu to the empty side. Cook for 5-7 minutes, stirring occasionally, until the tofu is heated through and lightly browned.
5. Mix the tofu with the vegetables in the skillet until well combined.
6. Serve hot and enjoy this flavorful and protein-rich turmeric scrambled tofu!

Nutrition Value (Per Serving)

Calories: 220 kcal - Carbohydrates: 10g - Protein: 14g - Fat: 15g - Fiber: 3g - Sugar: 3g - Sodium: 25mg

BREAKFAST QUINOA PORRIDGE WITH APPLE CINNAMON COMPOTE

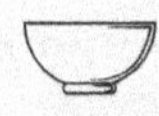 **Preparation Time : 5 min**

 **Cooking Time : 15 min**

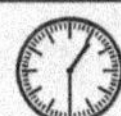 **Servings : 2**

Ingredients

- 1/2 cup quinoa, rinsed
- 1 cup almond milk
- 1 apple, peeled, cored, and diced
- 1 tablespoon maple syrup
- 1/2 teaspoon ground cinnamon
- Pinch of nutmeg
- Chopped nuts for garnish (optional)

Preparation

1. In a saucepan, combine quinoa and almond milk.
2. Bring to a boil, then reduce heat to low, cover, and simmer for 12-15 minutes, or until quinoa is cooked and liquid is absorbed.
3. In another saucepan, combine diced apple, maple syrup, ground cinnamon, and a pinch of nutmeg.
4. Cook over medium heat for 5-7 minutes, stirring occasionally, until the apples are tender and the mixture thickens slightly.
5. Divide the cooked quinoa into bowls.
6. Top each bowl with apple cinnamon compote.
7. Garnish with chopped nuts if desired.
8. Serve warm and enjoy this comforting and nutritious breakfast quinoa porridge!

Nutrition Value (Per Serving)

Calories: 250 kcal - Carbohydrates: 45g - Protein: 6g - Fat: 6g
- Fiber: 6g - Sugar: 14g - Sodium: 30mg

VEGETABLE FRITTATA

Preparation Time : 10 min

Cooking Time : 20 min

Servings : 2

Ingredients

- 4 large eggs
- 1 small zucchini, diced
- 1/2 bell pepper, diced
- 1/4 cup crumbled goat cheese
- Fresh herbs, optional garnish (parsley, basil, etc.)

Preparation

1. Preheat the oven to 350°F (175°C).
2. In a mixing bowl, whisk together eggs until well beaten. Set aside.
3. Heat a non-stick skillet over medium heat. Add diced zucchini and bell pepper, and cook until softened, about 5 minutes.
4. Pour beaten eggs over the cooked vegetables in the skillet.
5. Sprinkle crumbled goat cheese evenly over the eggs.
6. Cook for 3-5 minutes, or until the edges start to set.
7. Transfer the skillet to the preheated oven and bake for 10-12 minutes, or until the frittata is set and lightly golden on top.
8. Remove from the oven and let it cool for a few minutes before slicing.
9. Garnish with fresh herbs if desired.
10. Serve warm or at room temperature and enjoy this delicious and protein-rich vegetable frittata!

Nutrition Value (Per Serving)

Calories: 200 kcal- Carbohydrates: 5g - Protein: 14g- Fat: 14g- Fiber: 2g - Sugar: 3g- Sodium: 40mg

PROTEIN-PACKED SMOOTHIE BOWL

Preparation Time : 5 min

Cooking Time : 0 min

Servings : 1

Ingredients

- 1 cup fresh spinach
- 1 cup frozen pineapple chunks
- 1/2 cup almond milk
- 1 tablespoon hemp seeds
- Fresh fruit slices and additional hemp seeds for topping (optional)

Preparation

1. In a blender, combine fresh spinach, frozen pineapple chunks, almond milk, and hemp seeds.
2. Blend until smooth and creamy, adding more almond milk if needed to reach desired consistency.
3. Pour the smoothie into a bowl.
4. Top with fresh fruit slices and additional hemp seeds if desired.
5. Serve immediately and enjoy this refreshing and protein-packed smoothie bowl!

Nutrition Value (Per Serving)

Calories: 250 kcal - Carbohydrates: 35g - Protein: 8g - Fat: 10g - Fiber: 6g - Sugar: 20g - Sodium: 20mg

GLUTEN-FREE MUESLI

🥣 **Preparation Time : 5 min**

🍴 **Cooking Time : 0 min**

🕐 **Servings : 1**

Ingredients

- 1/2 cup gluten-free rolled oats
- 1/4 cup finely chopped nuts (almonds, pecans, or walnuts)
- 1 tablespoon chia seeds
- 1 tablespoon unsweetened shredded coconut
- 1/2 cup almond milk
- Fresh fruit slices for topping (such as berries or banana)

Preparation

1. In a bowl, combine gluten-free rolled oats, chopped nuts, chia seeds, and shredded coconut.
2. Pour almond milk over the dry ingredients and stir to combine.
3. Let the muesli sit for 5 minutes to allow the flavors to meld and the chia seeds to absorb some of the liquid.
4. Top with fresh fruit slices.
5. Serve immediately and enjoy this wholesome and satisfying gluten-free muesli!

Nutrition Value (Per Serving)

Calories: 300 kcal - Carbohydrates: 30g - Protein: 8g - Fat: 18g - Fiber: 8g - Sugar: 4g - Sodium: 20mg

Lunch Recipes

CHICKPEA NOODLE SOUP

Preparation Time : 10 min

Cooking Time : 24 min

Servings : 4

Ingredients

- 1 tablespoon olive oil
- 1 onion, diced
- 2 carrots, sliced
- 2 celery stalks, sliced
- 3 cloves garlic, minced
- 6 cups low-sodium vegetable broth
- 1 can (15 oz) chickpeas, drained and rinsed
- 1 cup uncooked chickpea noodles
- 1 teaspoon dried thyme
- 1 teaspoon dried oregano
- Salt and pepper to taste
- Fresh parsley for garnish (optional)

Preparation

1. In a big pot, warm up the olive oil over medium heat. Add diced onion, sliced carrots, and sliced celery. Cook until vegetables are softened, about 5-7 minutes.
2. Add the minced garlic and simmer for another 1-2 minutes, or until fragrant.
3. Pour in vegetable broth and bring to a simmer.
4. Add chickpeas, chickpea noodles, dried thyme, and dried oregano to the pot. Simmer for 10-12 minutes, or until noodles are cooked al dente.
5. Season with salt and pepper to taste.
6. Spoon soup into bowls; if desired, top with chopped fresh parsley.
7. Serve hot and enjoy this comforting and flavorful chickpea noodle soup!

Nutrition Value (Per Serving)

Calories: 280 kcal- Carbohydrates: 42g - Protein: 12g- Fat: 7g- Fiber: 10g - Sugar: 6g- Sodium: 30mg

VEGETABLE SOUP

Ingredients

- 1 tablespoon olive oil
- 1 onion, diced
- 2 carrots, sliced
- 2 celery stalks, sliced
- 1 bell pepper, diced
- 3 cloves garlic, minced
- 6 cups low-sodium vegetable broth
- 1 can (15 oz) diced tomatoes
- 1 cup chopped green beans
- 1 teaspoon dried thyme
- 1 teaspoon dried basil
- Salt and pepper to taste
- Fresh parsley for garnish (optional)

Preparation

1. In a big pot, warm up the olive oil over medium heat. Add diced onion, sliced carrots, sliced celery, diced bell pepper, and minced garlic.
2. Cook until vegetables are softened, about 5-7 minutes.
3. Pour in vegetable broth and diced tomatoes with their juices. Bring to a simmer.
4. Add chopped green beans, dried thyme, and dried basil to the pot.
5. Simmer for 10-12 minutes, or until vegetables are tender.
6. To taste, add salt and pepper for seasoning.
7. Ladle the soup into bowls and garnish with fresh parsley if desired.
8. Serve hot and enjoy this nutritious and satisfying vegetable soup!

Nutrition Value (Per Serving)

Calories: 150 kcal- Carbohydrates: 25g - Protein: 5g- Fat: 5g- Fiber: 6g
- Sugar: 9g- Sodium: 40mg

ZOODLE PAD THAI

Preparation Time : 15 min

Cooking Time : 10 min

Servings : 2

Ingredients

- 2 medium zucchinis, spiralized into noodles
- 1 tablespoon olive oil
- 2 cloves garlic, minced
- 1 red bell pepper, thinly sliced
- 2 carrots, julienned
- 1 cup bean sprouts
- 2 green onions, sliced
- 2 tablespoons chopped peanuts (optional, for garnish)
- Lime wedges for serving

For the Sauce:

- 3 tablespoons low-sodium soy sauce
- 1 tablespoon maple syrup or honey
- 1 tablespoon rice vinegar
- 1 tablespoon lime juice
- 1 teaspoon grated ginger
- 1 teaspoon sriracha (optional)

Preparation

1. In a small bowl, whisk together all the ingredients for the sauce. Set aside.
2. In a big skillet over medium heat, warm up the olive oil. Add the minced garlic and simmer for one minute, or until it becomes aromatic.
3. Add sliced bell pepper and julienned carrots to the skillet. Sauté the veggies for 3–4 minutes, or until they are crisp-tender.
4. Add zucchini noodles and bean sprouts to the skillet. Cook for 2-3 minutes until noodles are just tender.
5. Pour the sauce over the zucchini noodles and toss to coat evenly.
6. Remove from heat and garnish with sliced green onions and chopped peanuts if desired.
7. Serve hot, garnished with lime wedges.
8. Enjoy this healthy and flavorful zoodle Pad Thai!

Nutrition Value (Per Serving)

Calories: 180 kcal - Carbohydrates: 20g - Protein: 6g - Fat: 10g - Fiber: 5g - Sugar: 10g - Sodium: 20mg

SPINACH AND PEAR SALAD

Preparation Time : 10 min

Cooking Time : 0 min

Servings : 2

Ingredients

- 4 cups fresh spinach leaves
- 1 ripe pear, thinly sliced
- 2 tablespoons chopped walnuts
- 2 tablespoons dried cranberries
- 1 tablespoon balsamic vinegar
- 1 tablespoon olive oil
- Salt and pepper to taste

Preparation

1. In a large salad bowl, combine fresh spinach leaves, thinly sliced pear, chopped walnuts, and dried cranberries.
2. In a small bowl, whisk together balsamic vinegar, olive oil, salt, and pepper to make the dressing.
3. Drizzle the dressing over the salad, tossing gently to coat everything.
4. Serve immediately and enjoy this refreshing and nutritious spinach and pear salad!

Nutrition Value (Per Serving)

Calories: 180 kcal - Carbohydrates: 25g - Protein: 3g- Fat: 9g - Fiber: 6g - Sugar: 15g- Sodium: 20mg

ROASTED SWEET POTATO AND BLACK BEAN NACHOS

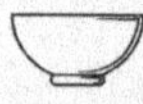 **Preparation Time : 10 min**

 **Cooking Time : 25 min**

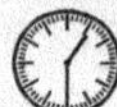 **Servings : 4**

Ingredients

- 2 medium sweet potatoes, peeled and thinly sliced
- 1 tablespoon olive oil
- 1 teaspoon ground cumin
- 1 teaspoon chili powder
- 1/2 teaspoon garlic powder
- Salt to taste
- 1 can (15 oz) black beans, drained and rinsed
- 1 cup shredded dairy-free cheese
- 1/4 cup chopped fresh cilantro
- Sliced jalapenos for garnish (optional)
- Dairy-free sour cream or salsa for serving (optional)

Preparation

1. Preheat the oven to 400°F (200°C). Line a baking sheet with parchment paper.
2. In a large bowl, toss sweet potato slices with olive oil, ground cumin, chili powder, garlic powder, and salt until evenly coated.
3. Arrange sweet potato slices in a single layer on the prepared baking sheet.
4. Roast in the preheated oven for 20-25 minutes, flipping halfway through, until sweet potatoes are tender and slightly crispy.
5. Remove from the oven and top sweet potato slices with black beans and shredded dairy-free cheese.
6. Return to the oven and bake for another 5 minutes, or until the cheese is melted and bubbly.
7. Remove from the oven and sprinkle with chopped fresh cilantro and sliced jalapenos if desired.
8. Serve hot with dairy-free sour cream or salsa on the side, if desired.
9. Enjoy these delicious and nutritious roasted sweet potato and black bean nachos!

Nutrition Value (Per Serving)

Calories: 280 kcal - Carbohydrates: 45g - Protein: 10g - Fat: 7g - Fiber: 10g - Sugar: 5g- Sodium: 30mg

ROASTED MEXICAN CAULIFLOWER

Preparation Time : 10 min

Cooking Time : 25 min

Servings : 4

Ingredients

- 1 head cauliflower, cut into florets
- 1 tablespoon olive oil
- 1 teaspoon ground cumin
- 1 teaspoon chili powder
- 1/2 teaspoon smoked paprika
- Salt and pepper to taste
- Fresh lime wedges for serving

Preparation

1. Preheat the oven to 425°F (220°C). Line a baking sheet with parchment paper.
2. In a large bowl, toss cauliflower florets with olive oil, ground cumin, chili powder, smoked paprika, salt, and pepper until evenly coated.
3. Spread cauliflower florets in a single layer on the prepared baking sheet.
4. Roast in the preheated oven for 20-25 minutes, flipping halfway through, until cauliflower is tender and lightly browned.
5. Remove from the oven and squeeze fresh lime juice over the roasted cauliflower.
6. Serve hot as a side dish or as part of your favorite Mexican-inspired meal.
7. Enjoy this flavorful and nutritious roasted Mexican cauliflower!

Nutrition Value (Per Serving)

Calories: 80 kcal - Carbohydrates: 10g - Protein: 3g - Fat: 4g - Fiber: 4g - Sugar: 4g - Sodium: 20mg

ROASTED BUTTERNUT SQUASH AND APPLE SOUP

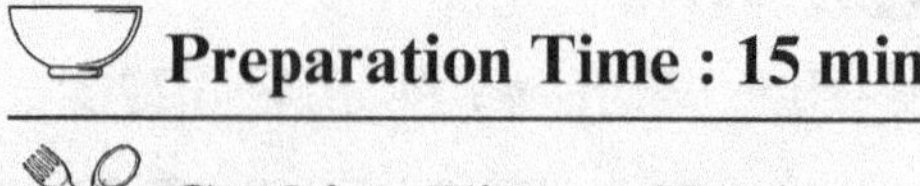

🥣 **Preparation Time : 15 min**

🍴 **Cooking Time : 45 min**

🕐 **Servings : 4**

Ingredients

- 1 medium butternut squash, peeled, seeded, and cubed
- 2 apples, peeled, cored, and diced
- 1 onion, chopped
- 2 cloves garlic, minced
- 4 cups low-sodium vegetable broth
- 1 teaspoon ground cinnamon
- 1/2 teaspoon ground nutmeg
- Salt and pepper to taste
- Fresh thyme for garnish (optional)

Preparation

1. Preheat the oven to 400°F (200°C). Line a baking sheet with parchment paper.
2. Place cubed butternut squash, diced apples, chopped onion, and minced garlic on the prepared baking sheet.
3. Drizzle with olive oil and toss to coat evenly. Add pepper, salt, and ground nutmeg along with the cinnamon.
4. Roast the vegetables for 30 to 35 minutes in a preheated oven, or until they are soft and have a light caramelization.
5. Transfer the roasted vegetables to a large pot. After adding the veggie broth, cook it.
6. Use an immersion blender to puree the soup until smooth. Alternatively, carefully transfer the soup in batches to a blender and blend until smooth, then return to the pot.
7. If necessary, add more salt and pepper for seasoning.
8. Ladle the soup into bowls and garnish with fresh thyme if desired.
9. Serve hot and enjoy this comforting and flavorful roasted butternut squash and apple soup!

Nutrition Value (Per Serving)

Calories: 150 kcal - Carbohydrates: 30g - Protein: 3g - Fat: 3g- Fiber: 6g
- Sugar: 12g - Sodium: 40mg

TURKEY BURGER

Preparation Time : 10 min

Cooking Time : 15 min

Servings : 4

Ingredients

- 1 lb. ground turkey
- 1/4 cup finely chopped onion
- 1 clove garlic, minced
- 1 tablespoon Worcestershire sauce
- 1 teaspoon dried oregano
- Salt and pepper to taste
- Lettuce leaves for serving
- Sliced tomatoes for serving
- Sliced avocado for serving
- Whole grain buns or lettuce wraps

Preparation

1. In a large bowl, combine ground turkey, chopped onion, minced garlic, Worcestershire sauce, dried oregano, salt, and pepper. Mix until well combined.
2. Divide the turkey mixture into 4 equal portions and shape each portion into a patty.
3. Heat a grill or skillet over medium heat.
4. Cook the turkey patties for 6-8 minutes on each side, or until fully cooked through and no longer pink in the center.
5. Serve the turkey burgers on whole grain buns or lettuce wraps, topped with lettuce leaves, sliced tomatoes, and sliced avocado.
6. Enjoy these juicy and flavorful turkey burgers as a delicious and low-sodium meal option!

Nutrition Value (Per Serving)

Calories: 250 kcal- Carbohydrates: 5g - Protein: 30g - Fat: 12g - Fiber: 1g - Sugar: 2g - Sodium: 40mg

PEAR AND WALNUT GRAIN SALAD

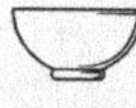 **Preparation Time : 10 min**

 **Cooking Time : 15 min**

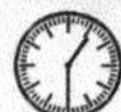 **Servings : 4**

Ingredients

- 1 cup of brown rice or cooked quinoa
- 2 ripe pears, diced
- 1/2 cup chopped walnuts
- 2 cups mixed salad greens
- 2 tablespoons balsamic vinegar
- 1 tablespoon olive oil
- Salt and pepper to taste

Preparation

1. In a large salad bowl, combine cooked quinoa or brown rice, diced pears, chopped walnuts, and mixed salad greens.
2. In a small bowl, whisk together balsamic vinegar, olive oil, salt, and pepper to make the dressing.
3. Drizzle the dressing over the salad, tossing gently to coat everything.
4. Serve immediately and enjoy this nutritious and flavorful pear and walnut grain salad!

Nutrition Value (Per Serving)

Calories: 200 kcal- Carbohydrates: 25g - Protein: 4g- Fat: 10g - Fiber: 5g - Sugar: 10g - Sodium: 20mg

VEGETABLE FRIED RICE

Preparation Time : 10 min

Cooking Time : 15 min

Servings : 4

Ingredients

- 2 cups cooked brown rice
- 1 cup mixed vegetables (such as peas, carrots, corn, and bell peppers)
- 2 cloves garlic, minced
- 2 tablespoons low-sodium soy sauce
- 1 tablespoon sesame oil
- 1 tablespoon rice vinegar
- 2 green onions, sliced
- Sesame seeds for garnish (optional)

Preparation

1. In a large skillet or wok, heat the sesame oil over medium heat. Cook for 1 minute, stirring in the minced garlic until fragrant.
2. Add mixed vegetables to the skillet and stir-fry for 3-4 minutes until tender.
3. Add cooked brown rice to the skillet and stir-fry for another 2-3 minutes to heat through.
4. In a small bowl, whisk together low-sodium soy sauce and rice vinegar. Pour the sauce over the rice and vegetables in the skillet.
5. Stir well to coat all the ingredients evenly with the sauce.
6. Take off the heat and, if you'd like, top with sesame seeds and chopped green onions.
7. Serve hot and enjoy this delicious and low-sodium vegetable fried rice!

Nutrition Value (Per Serving)

Calories: 220 kcal - Carbohydrates: 35g - Protein: 6g - Fat: 6g - Fiber: 5g - Sugar: 3g - Sodium: 30mg

VEGETABLE CURRY

🥣 **Preparation Time : 10 min**

🍴 **Cooking Time : 25 min**

🕐 **Servings : 4**

Ingredients

- 2 cups mixed vegetables (such as cauliflower, carrots, bell peppers, and green beans), chopped
- 1 onion, diced
- 2 cloves garlic, minced
- 1 tablespoon curry powder
- 1 can (14 oz) coconut milk
- 1 cup vegetable broth
- 1 tablespoon olive oil
- Salt and pepper to taste
- Fresh cilantro for garnish (optional)

Preparation

1. Heat olive oil in a large skillet or pot over medium heat. Add diced onion and minced garlic. Cook for 2-3 minutes until softened.
2. Add chopped mixed vegetables to the skillet and stir-fry for 5-6 minutes until slightly tender.
3. Sprinkle curry powder over the vegetables and stir to coat evenly.
4. Pour coconut milk and vegetable broth into the skillet. Stir well to combine.
5. Bring the mixture to a simmer and cook for 10-15 minutes, stirring occasionally, until the vegetables are cooked through and the curry sauce has thickened.
6. Season with salt and pepper to taste.
7. Serve hot, garnished with fresh cilantro if desired.
8. Enjoy this flavorful and nutritious vegetable curry as a satisfying low-sodium meal!

Nutrition Value (Per Serving)

Calories: 220 kcal - Carbohydrates: 15g - Protein: 5g - Fat: 17g - Fiber: 5g - Sugar: 7g - Sodium: 20mg

CUCUMBER SALAD

Preparation Time : 10 min

Cooking Time : 0 min

Servings : 4

Ingredients

- 2 cucumbers, thinly sliced
- 1/4 cup red onion, thinly sliced
- 2 tablespoons rice vinegar
- 1 tablespoon olive oil
- 1 teaspoon honey or maple syrup
- 1 tablespoon chopped fresh dill
- Salt and pepper to taste
- Sesame seeds for garnish (optional)

Preparation

1. In a large bowl, combine thinly sliced cucumbers and red onion.
2. In a small bowl, whisk together rice vinegar, olive oil, honey or maple syrup, chopped fresh dill, salt, and pepper to make the dressing.
3. Drizzle the dressing over the mixture of onions and cucumbers. In order to coat all the ingredients equally, gently toss.
4. Sprinkle sesame seeds over the salad for garnish if desired.
5. Serve immediately and enjoy this refreshing and flavorful cucumber salad!

Nutrition Value (Per Serving)

Calories: 40 kcal - Carbohydrates: 5g - Protein: 1g - Fat: 2g - Fiber: 1g - Sugar: 3g - Sodium: 20mg

FRIED TOFU

⌣ **Preparation Time : 10 min**

✕ **Cooking Time : 10 min**

🕐 **Servings : 2**

Ingredients

- 1 block (about 14 oz) firm tofu, drained and pressed
- 2 tablespoons cornstarch
- 1 tablespoon soy sauce
- 1 tablespoon rice vinegar
- 1 teaspoon maple syrup or honey
- 1 clove garlic, minced
- 1/2 teaspoon grated ginger
- 1 tablespoon sesame oil
- Sesame seeds for garnish (optional)
- Chopped green onions for garnish (optional)

Preparation

1. Cut the pressed tofu into cubes.
2. In a shallow dish, toss tofu cubes with cornstarch until evenly coated.
3. Heat sesame oil in a non-stick skillet over medium heat. Add tofu cubes and fry for 4-5 minutes on each side, or until golden brown and crispy.
4. In a small bowl, whisk together soy sauce, rice vinegar, maple syrup or honey, minced garlic, and grated ginger to make the sauce.
5. Pour the sauce over the fried tofu in the skillet. Toss gently to coat all the tofu cubes evenly with the sauce.
6. Remove from heat and garnish with sesame seeds and chopped green onions if desired.
7. Serve hot and enjoy this crispy and flavorful fried tofu!

Nutrition Value (Per Serving)

Calories: 200 kcal - Carbohydrates: 8g - Protein: 12g - Fat: 14g - Fiber: 2g - Sugar: 3g - Sodium: 40mg

THAI PRAWN SALAD

Preparation Time : 15 min

Cooking Time : 5 min

Servings : 2

Ingredients

- 8-10 large prawns, peeled and deveined
- 2 cups mixed salad greens
- 1/2 cucumber, thinly sliced
- 1/2 carrot, grated
- 1/4 cup chopped fresh cilantro
- 1/4 cup chopped fresh mint leaves
- 2 tablespoons chopped peanuts
- 1 tablespoon fish sauce
- 1 tablespoon lime juice
- 1 teaspoon honey or maple syrup
- 1 teaspoon grated ginger
- 1 clove garlic, minced
- Red chili flakes to taste (optional)

Preparation

1. Heat a grill or skillet over medium-high heat.
2. Cook prawns for 2-3 minutes on each side, or until cooked through and pink.
3. In a large bowl, combine mixed salad greens, thinly sliced cucumber, grated carrot, chopped fresh cilantro, chopped fresh mint leaves, and chopped peanuts.
4. In a small bowl, whisk together fish sauce, lime juice, honey or maple syrup, grated ginger, minced garlic, and red chili flakes to make the dressing.
5. Add cooked prawns to the salad bowl and drizzle the dressing over the salad.
6. Gently toss to ensure that the dressing coats every ingredient equally.
7. Serve immediately and enjoy this vibrant and flavorful Thai prawn salad!

Nutrition Value (Per Serving)

Calories: 180 kcal - Carbohydrates: 10g - Protein: 15g - Fat: 8g - Fiber: 3g - Sugar: 5g - Sodium: 50mg

SWEET CORN AND BLACK BEAN TACOS

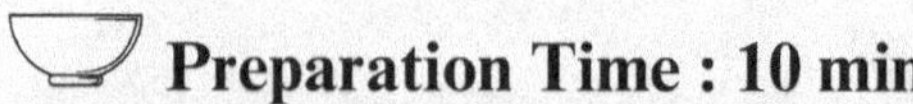 **Preparation Time : 10 min**

Cooking Time : 10 min

Servings : 2

Ingredients

- 4 small corn tortillas
- 1 cup canned black beans, drained and rinsed
- 1 cup cooked sweet corn kernels
- 1/2 avocado, sliced
- 1/4 cup salsa
- 2 tablespoons chopped fresh cilantro
- Lime wedges for serving

Preparation

1. Heat corn tortillas in a skillet over medium heat for 1-2 minutes on each side, or until warmed through.
2. In a small saucepan, heat black beans and sweet corn kernels until warmed.
3. Assemble tacos by layering black beans, sweet corn kernels, sliced avocado, salsa, and chopped fresh cilantro on each corn tortilla.
4. Serve with lime wedges on the side.
5. Enjoy these delicious and satisfying sweet corn and black bean tacos as a flavorful and low-sodium meal option!

Nutrition Value (Per Serving)

Calories: 220 kcal - Carbohydrates: 35g - Protein: 8g - Fat: 7g - Fiber: 8g
- Sugar: 5g - Sodium: 40mg

MINESTRONE SOUP

Preparation Time : 15 min

Cooking Time : 25 min

Servings : 4

Ingredients

- 4 cups low-sodium vegetable broth
- 1 can (14 oz) diced tomatoes
- 1 cup chopped carrots
- 1 cup chopped celery
- 1 cup chopped zucchini
- 1 cup cooked small pasta (such as elbow or shell)
- 1 can (15 oz) of washed and drained kidney beans
- 2 cloves garlic, minced
- 1 teaspoon dried oregano
- 1 teaspoon dried basil
- Salt and pepper to taste
- Fresh parsley for garnish (optional)

Preparation

1. In a large pot, combine vegetable broth, diced tomatoes (with their juices), chopped carrots, chopped celery, minced garlic, dried oregano, and dried basil.
2. Bring the mixture to a boil, then reduce heat to low and let it simmer for 15 minutes, stirring occasionally.
3. Add chopped zucchini, cooked pasta, and kidney beans to the pot. Simmer for an additional 5-10 minutes until the vegetables are soft.
4. Season with salt and pepper to taste.
5. Ladle the soup into bowls and garnish with fresh parsley if desired.
6. Serve hot and enjoy this hearty and flavorful minestrone soup!

Nutrition Value (Per Serving)

Calories: 180 kcal - Carbohydrates: 35g - Protein: 8g - Fat: 1g - Fiber: 8g - Sugar: 6g - Sodium: 40mg

VEGGIE SUSHI ROLLS

Preparation Time : 20 min

Cooking Time : 20 min

Servings : 2

Ingredients

- 2 nori seaweed sheets
- 1 cup cooked quinoa
- 1 avocado, thinly sliced
- 1/2 cucumber, julienned
- 1/2 carrot, julienned
- 2 tablespoons rice vinegar
- 1 teaspoon sugar
- Pinch of salt
- Soy sauce and wasabi for serving (optional)

Preparation

1. In a small bowl, mix cooked quinoa with rice vinegar, sugar, and a pinch of salt. Allow it to cool slightly.
2. Place a nori seaweed sheet on a bamboo sushi mat or a clean kitchen towel.
3. Spread half of the cooked quinoa evenly over the nori sheet, leaving about 1 inch of space at the top.
4. Arrange avocado slices, cucumber, and carrot strips horizontally on top of the quinoa.
5. Roll the sushi tightly using the bamboo mat or towel, pressing gently as you roll to seal.
6. Repeat the process with the second nori sheet and remaining ingredients.
7. Use a sharp knife to slice each roll into 6-8 pieces.
8. Serve with soy sauce and wasabi on the side if desired.
9. Enjoy these delicious and nutritious veggie sushi rolls with quinoa and avocado!

Nutrition Value (Per Serving)

Calories: 250 kcal - Carbohydrates: 35g - Protein: 6g - Fat: 10g - Fiber: 8g - Sugar: 2g - Sodium: 20mg

MEDITERRANEAN CHICKPEA STEW

Preparation Time : 15 min

Cooking Time : 25 min

Servings : 4

Ingredients

- 2 tablespoons olive oil
- 1 onion, diced
- 2 cloves garlic, minced
- 1 teaspoon ground cumin
- 1 teaspoon ground coriander
- 1/2 teaspoon smoked paprika
- 1 can (15 oz) chickpeas, drained and rinsed
- 1 can (14 oz) diced tomatoes
- 2 cups vegetable broth
- 2 cups fresh spinach leaves
- 1/4 cup sliced black olives
- Salt and pepper to taste
- Fresh parsley for garnish (optional)

Preparation

1. In a large pot, heat the olive oil over medium heat. Add diced onion and minced garlic. Cook for 2-3 minutes until softened.
2. Add ground cumin, ground coriander, and smoked paprika to the pot. Stir thoroughly to coat the onions and garlic in the seasonings.
3. Add chickpeas, diced tomatoes (with their juices), and vegetable broth to the pot.
4. Bring to a boil, then cook for 15-20 minutes, stirring regularly.
5. Stir in fresh spinach leaves and sliced black olives.
6. Cook for another 2-3 minutes until the spinach wilts.
7. Season with salt and pepper to taste.
8. Ladle the stew into bowls and garnish with fresh parsley if desired.
9. Serve hot and enjoy this flavorful and hearty Mediterranean chickpea stew!

Nutrition Value (Per Serving)

Calories: 200 kcal - Carbohydrates: 25g - Protein: 8g - Fat: 8g - Fiber: 8g - Sugar: 5g - Sodium: 30mg

LENTIL SOUP

🥣 **Preparation Time : 10 min**

🍴 **Cooking Time : 30 min**

🕐 **Servings : 4**

Ingredients

- 1 cup dried lentils, rinsed
- 4 cups low-sodium vegetable broth
- 1 onion, diced
- 2 carrots, diced
- 2 celery stalks, diced
- 2 cloves garlic, minced
- 2 cups chopped kale leaves
- 1 teaspoon ground turmeric
- 1 teaspoon ground cumin
- Salt and pepper to taste
- Fresh lemon juice for serving (optional)
- Fresh parsley for garnish (optional)

Preparation

1. In a large pot, combine dried lentils and vegetable broth.
2. Bring to a boil, then reduce heat to low and let it simmer for 15 minutes.
3. Add diced onion, diced carrots, diced celery, and minced garlic to the pot.
4. Continue to simmer for another 10-15 minutes, or until the lentils and vegetables are tender.
5. Stir in chopped kale leaves, ground turmeric, and ground cumin.
6. Simmer for an additional 5 minutes until the kale is wilted.
7. Season with salt and pepper to taste.
8. Serve hot, squeezing fresh lemon juice over each serving if desired, and garnish with fresh parsley.
9. Enjoy this nutritious and flavorful lentil soup with kale and turmeric!

Nutrition Value (Per Serving)

Calories: 200 kcal - Carbohydrates: 35g - Protein: 12g - Fat: 1g - Fiber: 12g - Sugar: 5g - Sodium: 40mg

STUFFED BELL PEPPERS

🥣 **Preparation Time : 15 min**

🍴 **Cooking Time : 35 min**

🕐 **Servings : 4**

Ingredients

- 4 Large bell peppers, half with seeds removed.
- 1 lb. lean ground turkey
- 1 cup cooked brown rice
- 1 onion, diced
- 2 cloves garlic, minced
- 1 teaspoon dried oregano
- 1 teaspoon dried basil
- 1 can (14 oz) chopped tomatoes, drained
- Salt and pepper to taste
- Fresh parsley for garnish (optional)

Preparation

1. Preheat the oven to 375°F (190°C).
2. Arrange halved bell peppers in a baking dish.
3. In a skillet, cook ground turkey over medium heat until browned.
4. Add the minced garlic and onion, and sauté until the ingredients are tender.
5. Stir in cooked brown rice, dried oregano, dried basil, and diced tomatoes.
6. Season with salt and pepper to taste.
7. Spoon the turkey and rice mixture into each bell pepper half, pressing gently to fill.
8. Cover the baking dish with foil and bake in the preheated oven for 25-30 minutes, or until the peppers are tender.
9. Remove from the oven and garnish with fresh parsley if desired.
10. Serve hot and enjoy these delicious stuffed bell peppers with ground turkey and brown rice!

Nutrition Value (Per Serving)

Calories: 250 kcal - Carbohydrates: 25g - Protein: 20g - Fat: 8g - Fiber: 6g - Sugar: 8g - Sodium: 30mg

TUNA SALAD

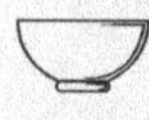 **Preparation Time : 10 min**

 **Cooking Time : 0 min**

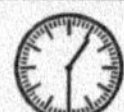 **Servings : 2**

Ingredients

- 1 can (5 oz) tuna, drained
- 1/4 cup Greek yogurt
- 1 tablespoon chopped fresh dill
- 1/4 cup diced cucumber
- 1/4 cup diced red bell pepper
- 1/4 cup diced red onion
- Salt and pepper to taste
- 4 large leaves of lettuce (iceberg or romaine)

Preparation

1. In a bowl, combine drained tuna, Greek yogurt, chopped fresh dill, diced cucumber, diced red bell pepper, and diced red onion.
2. Season with salt and pepper to taste.
3. Mix thoroughly to mix all of the ingredients.
4. Spoon the tuna salad mixture onto each lettuce leaf.
5. Roll up the lettuce leaves to form wraps.
6. Serve immediately and enjoy these light and refreshing tuna salad lettuce wraps with Greek yogurt and dill!

Nutrition Value (Per Serving)

Calories: 150 kcal - Carbohydrates: 6g - Protein: 20g - Fat: 5g - Fiber: 2g - Sugar: 3g - Sodium: 20mg

TURKEY AND VEGETABLE STIR-FRY WITH BROWN RICE

🥣 **Preparation Time : 5 min**

🍴 **Cooking Time : 15 min**

🕐 **Servings : 4**

Ingredients

- 1 lb. turkey breast, thinly sliced
- 2 cups of sliced mixed veggies, including bell peppers, broccoli, carrots, and snap peas
- 2 cloves garlic, minced
- 1 tablespoon low-sodium soy sauce
- 1 tablespoon olive oil
- 1 teaspoon grated ginger
- 2 cups cooked brown rice
- Salt and pepper to taste
- Sesame seeds for garnish (optional)
- Chopped green onions for garnish (optional)

Preparation

1. In a large skillet or wok, heat the olive oil over medium-high heat.
2. Add minced garlic and grated ginger. Cook for 1 minute until fragrant.
3. Add thinly sliced turkey breast to the skillet.
4. Stir-fry for an additional 3-4 minutes, or until the vegetables are soft and crispy.
5. Add sliced mixed vegetables to the skillet.
6. Stir-fry for another 3-4 minutes until the vegetables are tender-crisp.
7. Stir in low-sodium soy sauce and cooked brown rice.
8. Cook for 2-3 minutes to heat through.
9. Season with salt and pepper to taste.
10. Serve hot, garnished with sesame seeds and chopped green onions if desired.
11. Enjoy this delicious and nutritious turkey and vegetable stir-fry with brown rice!

Nutrition Value (Per Serving)

Calories: 250 kcal - Carbohydrates: 25g - Protein: 25g - Fat: 6g - Fiber: 4g - Sugar: 3g - Sodium: 30mg

QUINOA SALAD

🥣 **Preparation Time : 25 min**

🍴 **Cooking Time : 15 min**

🕐 **Servings : 4**

Ingredients

- 1 cup quinoa, rinsed
- 2 cups chopped mixed vegetables (include red onion, bell peppers, zucchini, and cherry tomatoes)
- 2 tablespoons olive oil
- Salt and pepper to taste
- 1/4 cup tahini
- 2 tablespoons fresh lemon juice
- 1 clove garlic, minced
- 1 tablespoon chopped fresh parsley
- Water for thinning the dressing

Preparation

1. Preheat the oven to 400°F (200°C). Line a baking sheet with parchment paper.
2. In a bowl, toss chopped mixed vegetables with olive oil, salt, and pepper until evenly coated.
3. Arrange the vegetables on the prepared baking sheet in a single layer. Roast in the preheated oven for 20-25 minutes, stirring halfway through, until tender and lightly browned.
4. In a small bowl, whisk together tahini, fresh lemon juice, minced garlic, chopped fresh parsley, and water until smooth and creamy. To get the right consistency, add water as needed.
5. Cook quinoa according to package instructions. Fluff with a fork and let it cool slightly.
6. Toss the cooked quinoa with the roasted veggies and the lemon-tahini dressing in a large bowl. Gently toss to evenly coat all of the ingredients.
7. Serve the quinoa salad warm or at room temperature.
8. Enjoy this flavorful and nutritious quinoa salad with roasted vegetables and lemon tahini dressing!

Nutrition Value (Per Serving)

Calories: 220 kcal - Carbohydrates: 30g - Protein: 6g - Fat: 10g - Fiber: 5g - Sugar: 3g - Sodium: 20mg

Dinner Recipes

BLACK BEANS QUESADILLA

🥣 **Preparation Time : 10 min**

🍴 **Cooking Time : 10 min**

🕐 **Servings : 2**

Ingredients

- 4 small whole wheat tortillas
- 1 cup cooked black beans
- 1/2 cup shredded cheddar cheese
- 1/4 cup diced tomatoes
- 1/4 cup diced red onion
- 1/4 cup chopped fresh cilantro
- 1 teaspoon ground cumin
- 1/2 teaspoon chili powder
- 1 tablespoon olive oil
- Salt and pepper to taste
- Salsa and Greek yogurt for serving (optional)

Preparation

1. In a bowl, mash the cooked black beans with ground cumin, chili powder, salt, and pepper.
2. Spread the mashed black beans evenly onto two tortillas.
3. Sprinkle shredded cheddar cheese over the black beans.
4. Top with diced tomatoes, diced red onion, and chopped fresh cilantro.
5. Place the remaining tortillas on top to form quesadillas.
6. Heat olive oil in a skillet over medium heat.
7. Cook each quesadilla for two to three minutes on each side, or until crispy and golden brown.
8. Remove from the skillet and cut each quesadilla into wedges.
9. Serve hot with salsa and Greek yogurt on the side if desired.
10. Enjoy these delicious and satisfying black beans quesadillas!

Nutrition Value (Per Serving)

Calories: 350 kcal - Carbohydrates: 40g - Protein: 15g - Fat: 15g - Fiber: 10g - Sugar: 2g - Sodium: 40mg

BROCCOLI CHEDDAR FRITTATA

Preparation Time : 10 min

Cooking Time : 20 min

Servings : 4

Ingredients

- 6 large eggs
- 1 cup chopped broccoli florets
- 1/2 cup shredded cheddar cheese
- 1/4 cup diced onion
- 1 clove garlic, minced
- 2 tablespoons chopped fresh parsley
- 1 tablespoon olive oil
- Salt and pepper to taste

Preparation

1. Preheat the oven to 350°F (175°C).
2. In a bowl, whisk together eggs, salt, and pepper until well beaten.
3. Heat olive oil in an oven-safe skillet over medium heat.
4. Add diced onion and minced garlic. Cook until tender, about 3–4 minutes more.
5. Add chopped broccoli florets to the skillet. Cook for another 3-4 minutes until tender.
6. Pour the beaten eggs into the skillet, covering the broccoli and onion evenly.
7. Sprinkle shredded cheddar cheese over the top.
8. Transfer the skillet to the preheated oven and bake for 15-20 minutes until the frittata is set and golden brown on top.
9. Remove from the oven and sprinkle chopped fresh parsley over the frittata.
10. Slice into wedges and serve hot or at room temperature.
11. Enjoy this delicious and nutritious broccoli cheddar frittata!

Nutrition Value (Per Serving)

Calories: 200 kcal - Carbohydrates: 5g - Protein: 15g - Fat: 15g - Fiber: 2g - Sugar: 2g - Sodium: 30mg

ASIAN SESAME SALMON

⬤ **Preparation Time : 10 min**

⬤ **Cooking Time : 15 min**

⬤ **Servings : 2**

Ingredients

- 2 salmon fillets
- 2 tablespoons low-sodium soy sauce
- 1 tablespoon sesame oil
- 1 tablespoon honey
- 1 tablespoon rice vinegar
- 1 clove garlic, minced
- 1 teaspoon grated ginger
- 1 tablespoon sesame seeds
- Sliced green onions for garnish
- Cooked brown rice for serving

Preparation

1. Preheat the oven to 400°F (200°C).
2. Line a baking sheet with parchment paper.
3. In a small bowl, whisk together low-sodium soy sauce, sesame oil, honey, rice vinegar, minced garlic, and grated ginger to make the marinade.
4. 3.Put the salmon fillets onto the baking sheet that has been prepared.
5. Pour the marinade over the salmon, coating each fillet evenly.
6. Sprinkle sesame seeds over the salmon.
7. Bake the salmon for 12 to 15 minutes, or until it is cooked through and flake readily with a fork, in the preheated oven
8. Remove from the oven and garnish with sliced green onions.
9. Serve hot with cooked brown rice.
10. Enjoy this flavorful and healthy Asian sesame salmon!

Nutrition Value (Per Serving)

Calories: 300 kcal - Carbohydrates: 10g - Protein: 25g - Fat: 15g - Fiber: 1g - Sugar: 8g - Sodium: 30mg

ONE POT CHICKEN AND RICE PILAF

Preparation Time : 10 min

Cooking Time : 30 min

Servings : 4

Ingredients

- 1 lb. boneless, skinless chicken breasts, cut into bite-sized pieces
- 1 cup long-grain white rice
- 2 cups low-sodium chicken broth
- 1 onion, diced
- 2 cloves garlic, minced
- 1 bell pepper, diced
- 1 carrot, diced
- 1 cup frozen peas
- 1 teaspoon ground cumin
- 1 teaspoon paprika
- 1/2 teaspoon turmeric
- Salt and pepper to taste
- Fresh parsley for garnish (optional)

Preparation

1. Heat some olive oil in a big pot over medium heat.
2. Add diced onion, minced garlic, diced bell pepper, and diced carrot. Cook until softened, about 5 minutes.
3. Add the bite-sized chicken pieces to the pot and cook until browned on all sides, about 5 minutes.
4. Stir in the long-grain white rice, ground cumin, paprika, turmeric, salt, and pepper.
5. Cook for another 2 minutes to toast the rice and spices.
6. Pour in the low-sodium chicken broth and bring to a boil.
7. Reduce the heat to low, cover the pot, and simmer for 15-20 minutes, or until the rice is cooked and the liquid is absorbed.
8. Stir in the frozen peas and let them heat through for a couple of minutes.
9. Garnish with fresh parsley if desired before serving.
10. Serve hot and enjoy this flavorful one-pot chicken and rice pilaf!

Nutrition Value (Per Serving)

Calories: 300 kcal - Carbohydrates: 35g - Protein: 25g - Fat: 6g - Fiber: 3g - Sugar: 3g - Sodium: 40mg

ITALIAN ARUGULA SALAD

Preparation Time : 10 min

Cooking Time : 0 min

Servings : 4

Ingredients

- 4 cups arugula
- 1 cup cherry tomatoes, halved
- 1/4 cup sliced black olives
- 1/4 cup diced red onion
- 2 tablespoons extra virgin olive oil
- 1 tablespoon balsamic vinegar
- 1 teaspoon Dijon mustard
- Salt and pepper to taste
- Shaved Parmesan cheese for garnish (optional)

Preparation

1. In a large salad bowl, combine arugula, cherry tomatoes, sliced black olives, and diced red onion.
2. To make the dressing, combine the extra virgin olive oil, dijon mustard, balsamic vinegar, salt, and pepper in a small bowl.
3. Drizzle the dressing over the salad and toss gently to coat all the ingredients evenly.
4. Garnish with shaved Parmesan cheese if desired.
5. Serve immediately and enjoy this refreshing Italian arugula salad!

Nutrition Value (Per Serving)

Calories: 120 kcal - Carbohydrates: 8g - Protein: 2g - Fat: 10g - Fiber: 2g - Sugar: 3g - Sodium: 30mg

CURRY CORN CHOWDER

🥣 **Preparation Time : 10 min**

🍴 **Cooking Time : 25 min**

🕐 **Servings : 4**

Ingredients

- 2 cups fresh or frozen corn kernels
- 1 potato, diced
- 1 onion, diced
- 2 cloves garlic, minced
- 2 cups low-sodium vegetable broth
- 1 cup coconut milk
- 1 teaspoon curry powder
- 1/2 teaspoon ground cumin
- 1/2 teaspoon ground turmeric
- Salt and pepper to taste
- Chopped fresh cilantro for garnish (optional)

Preparation

1. In a large pot, combine fresh or frozen corn kernels, diced potato, diced onion, minced garlic, low-sodium vegetable broth, coconut milk, curry powder, ground cumin, ground turmeric, salt, and pepper.
2. Bring the mixture to a boil, then reduce heat to low and simmer for 20-25 minutes, or until the vegetables are tender.
3. Use an immersion blender to blend the soup until smooth and creamy. Alternatively, put the soup in a blender and process it in batches until it becomes smooth.
4. Adjust seasoning with more salt and pepper if needed.
5. Ladle the curry corn chowder into bowls and garnish with chopped fresh cilantro if desired.
6. Serve hot and enjoy this comforting and flavorful curry corn chowder!

Nutrition Value (Per Serving)

Calories: 200 kcal - Carbohydrates: 25g - Protein: 3g - Fat: 10g - Fiber: 4g - Sugar: 5g - Sodium: 40mg

PAN-ROASTED MACKEREL WITH VEGETABLES

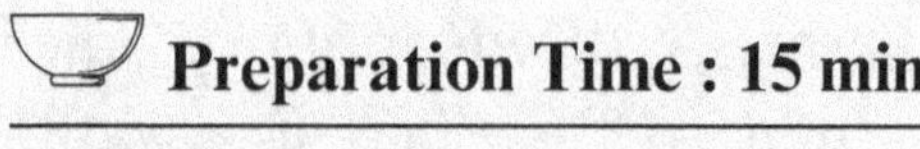

🥣 **Preparation Time : 15 min**

🍴 **Cooking Time : 20 min**

🕐 **Servings : 2**

Ingredients

- 2 mackerel fillets
- 2 cups chopped mixed vegetables (include red onion, bell peppers, zucchini, and cherry tomatoes)
- 2 tablespoons olive oil
- 1 tablespoon lemon juice
- 2 cloves garlic, minced
- Salt and pepper to taste
- Fresh herbs for garnish (optional)

Preparation

1. Preheat the oven to 400°F (200°C).
2. In a bowl, toss the mixed vegetables with olive oil, lemon juice, minced garlic, salt, and pepper until evenly coated.
3. Arrange the seasoned veggies in a single layer on a baking pan.
4. Place the mackerel fillets on top of the vegetables.
5. Roast in the preheated oven for 15-20 minutes, or until the mackerel is cooked through and flakes easily with a fork.
6. Remove from the oven and garnish with fresh herbs if desired.
7. Serve hot and enjoy this delicious and nutritious pan-roasted mackerel with vegetables!

Nutrition Value (Per Serving)

Calories: 250 kcal - Carbohydrates: 10g - Protein: 20g - Fat: 15g - Fiber: 3g - Sugar: 5g - Sodium: 30mg

FALAFEL SESAME BOWL

🥣 **Preparation Time : 15 min**

🍴 **Cooking Time : 15 min**

🕐 **Servings : 2**

Ingredients

- 8 falafel balls
- 2 cups cooked quinoa
- 1 cup mixed greens (such as spinach, kale, and arugula)
- 1/2 cucumber, sliced
- 1/2 cup cherry tomatoes, halved
- 1/4 cup sliced red onion
- 2 tablespoons tahini
- 1 tablespoon lemon juice
- 1 tablespoon water
- 1 tablespoon sesame seeds
- Salt and pepper to taste

Preparation

1. Cook the falafel balls according to package instructions until crispy and golden brown.
2. In a bowl, combine cooked quinoa, mixed greens, sliced cucumber, halved cherry tomatoes, and sliced red onion.
3. In a small bowl, whisk together tahini, lemon juice, water, salt, and pepper to make the dressing.
4. Divide the quinoa and vegetable mixture between two bowls.
5. Top each bowl with falafel balls and drizzle with the tahini dressing.
6. Sprinkle sesame seeds over the bowls.
7. Serve immediately and enjoy this flavorful and satisfying falafel sesame bowl!

Nutrition Value (Per Serving)

Calories: 350 kcal - Carbohydrates: 40g - Protein: 15g - Fat: 15g - Fiber: 8g - Sugar: 5g - Sodium: 40mg

GINGER AND GREENS SOUP

🥣 **Preparation Time : 10 min**

🍴 **Cooking Time : 20 min**

🕐 **Servings : 4**

Ingredients

- 4 cups vegetable broth
- 2 cups mixed greens (such as spinach, kale, and Swiss chard), chopped
- 1 onion, diced
- 2 cloves garlic, minced
- 1 tablespoon grated ginger
- 1 tablespoon olive oil
- Salt and pepper to taste
- Sliced green onions for garnish (optional)

Preparation

1. In a big pot, warm up the olive oil over medium heat.
2. Add diced onion and minced garlic. Cook until softened, about 5 minutes.
3. Add grated ginger to the pot and cook for another 1-2 minutes until fragrant.
4. Pour vegetable broth into the pot and bring to a simmer.
5. Add chopped mixed greens to the pot. Cook for 10-15 minutes until the greens are wilted and tender.
6. Blend the soup with an immersion blender until it's smooth. Alternately, transfer the soup to a blender and blend in batches until smooth.
7. Season with salt and pepper to taste.
8. Ladle the ginger and greens soup into bowls.
9. Garnish with sliced green onions if desired.
10. Serve hot and enjoy this comforting and nutritious soup!

Nutrition Value (Per Serving)

Calories: 100 kcal - Carbohydrates: 10g - Protein: 3g - Fat: 6g - Fiber: 3g - Sugar: 4g - Sodium: 30mg

SUPER GREEN SOUP

🥣 **Preparation Time : 10 min**

🍴 **Cooking Time : 25 min**

🕐 **Servings : 4**

Ingredients

- 4 cups low-sodium vegetable broth
- 2 cups mixed greens (such as spinach, kale, and broccoli), chopped
- 1 cup frozen peas
- 1 onion, diced
- 2 cloves garlic, minced
- 1 tablespoon olive oil
- 1 tablespoon lemon juice
- Salt and pepper to taste
- Sliced avocado for garnish (optional)

Preparation

1. In a big pot, warm up the olive oil over medium heat. Add diced onion and minced garlic. Cook until softened, about 5 minutes.
2. Pour vegetable broth into the pot and bring to a simmer.
3. Add chopped mixed greens and frozen peas to the pot.
4. Cook for 10-15 minutes until the greens are wilted and the peas are heated through.
5. Blend the soup with an immersion blender until it's smooth. Or put the soup in a blender and process in batches until smooth.
6. Stir in lemon juice and season with salt and pepper to taste.
7. Ladle the super green soup into bowls.
8. Garnish with sliced avocado if desired.
9. Serve hot and enjoy this vibrant and nutritious soup!

Nutrition Value (Per Serving)

Calories: 120 kcal - Carbohydrates: 12g - Protein: 4g - Fat: 6g - Fiber: 4g - Sugar: 4g - Sodium: 40mg

KALE, SMOKED TROUT AND AVOCADO SALAD

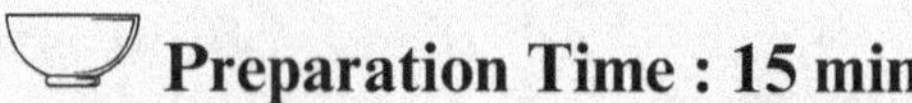

🥣 **Preparation Time : 15 min**

🍴 **Cooking Time : 0 min**

🕐 **Servings : 2**

Ingredients

- 4 cups kale, chopped
- 1 smoked trout fillet, flaked
- 1 avocado, sliced
- 1/4 cup sliced almonds
- 1/4 cup dried cranberries
- 2 tablespoons olive oil
- 1 tablespoon lemon juice
- 1 teaspoon Dijon mustard
- Salt and pepper to taste

Preparation

1. In a large bowl, combine chopped kale, flaked smoked trout, sliced avocado, sliced almonds, and dried cranberries.
2. In a small bowl, whisk together olive oil, lemon juice, Dijon mustard, salt, and pepper to make the dressing.
3. Drizzle the dressing over the salad and toss gently to coat all the ingredients evenly.
4. Serve immediately and enjoy this nutritious and flavorful kale, smoked trout, and avocado salad!

Nutrition Value (Per Serving)

Calories: 300 kcal - Carbohydrates: 20g - Protein: 15g - Fat: 20g - Fiber: 8g - Sugar: 6g - Sodium: 40mg

TURKEY MEATBALLS ZUCCHINI NOODLES

Preparation Time : 20 min

Cooking Time : 25 min

Servings : 2

Ingredients

- 8 oz ground turkey
- 1/4 cup breadcrumbs
- 1 egg
- 2 cloves garlic, minced
- 1/4 cup grated Parmesan cheese
- 2 cups marinara sauce (low-sodium)
- 2 medium zucchinis, spiralized into noodles
- 1 tablespoon olive oil
- Salt and pepper to taste
- Fresh basil leaves for garnish (optional)

Preparation

1. In a bowl, combine ground turkey, breadcrumbs, egg, minced garlic, and grated Parmesan cheese. Season with salt and pepper. Mix until well combined.
2. Roll the turkey mixture into meatballs, about 1 inch in diameter.
3. In a big skillet, warm up the olive oil over medium heat. Add the turkey meatballs and cook for 5-7 minutes, turning occasionally, until browned on all sides.
4. Pour marinara sauce into the skillet, covering the meatballs. Reduce heat to low, cover, and simmer for 15 minutes, or until the meatballs are cooked through.
5. While the meatballs are simmering, heat olive oil in another skillet over medium heat. Add spiralized zucchini noodles and cook for 2-3 minutes until tender-crisp.
6. Serve the turkey meatballs in marinara sauce over the zucchini noodles.
7. Garnish with fresh basil leaves if desired.
8. Enjoy this light and flavorful dish of turkey meatballs in marinara sauce with zucchini noodles!

Nutrition Value (Per Serving)

Calories: 300 kcal - Carbohydrates: 20g - Protein: 25g - Fat: 15g - Fiber: 5g - Sugar: 10g - Sodium: 30mg

GRILLED VEGETABLE AND CHICKPEA SALAD

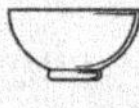 **Preparation Time : 15 min**

 **Cooking Time : 15 min**

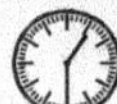 **Servings : 4**

Ingredients

- 2 cups mixed vegetables (such as bell peppers, zucchini, eggplant, and cherry tomatoes), sliced
- 1 can (15 oz) chickpeas, drained and rinsed
- 2 tablespoons olive oil
- Salt and pepper to taste
- 4 cups mixed greens (such as spinach, arugula, and lettuce)
- 1/4 cup chopped fresh parsley
- 1 lemon, juiced
- 2 tablespoons extra virgin olive oil

Preparation

1. Preheat the grill to medium-high heat.
2. In a bowl, toss the mixed vegetables and chickpeas with olive oil, salt, and pepper until evenly coated.
3. Grill the vegetables and chickpeas for 8-10 minutes, turning occasionally, until charred and tender.
4. In a large salad bowl, combine the grilled vegetables and chickpeas with mixed greens and chopped fresh parsley.
5. In a small bowl, whisk together lemon juice and extra virgin olive oil to make the vinaigrette.
6. Drizzle the lemon vinaigrette over the salad and toss gently to coat.
7. Serve immediately and enjoy this refreshing and nutritious grilled vegetable and chickpea salad!

Nutrition Value (Per Serving)

Calories: 250 kcal- Carbohydrates: 25g - Protein: 8g - Fat: 15g - Fiber: 6g - Sugar: 4g - Sodium: 30mg

BAKED SALMON WITH DILL SAUCE AND ROASTED ASPARAGUS

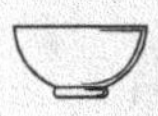 **Preparation Time : 10 min**

 **Cooking Time : 20 min**

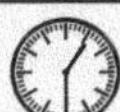 **Servings : 2**

Ingredients

- 2 salmon filets
- 1 bunch asparagus, trimmed
- 1 tablespoon olive oil
- Salt and pepper to taste
- 1 tablespoon fresh dill, chopped
- 1/4 cup Greek yogurt
- 1 tablespoon lemon juice
- 1 teaspoon Dijon mustard

Preparation

1. Preheat the oven to 400°F (200°C).
2. Arrange the salmon fillets onto a parchment paper-lined baking sheet. Season with salt, pepper, and chopped fresh dill.
3. Arrange the trimmed asparagus on the same baking sheet. Sprinkle with salt and pepper and drizzle with olive oil.
4. Bake in the preheated oven for 15-20 minutes, or until the salmon is cooked through and flakes easily with a fork, and the asparagus is tender.
5. Combine Greek yogurt, lemon juice, Dijon mustard, and a small pinch of salt in a small bowl and whisk until smooth.
6. Serve the baked salmon and roasted asparagus with the dill sauce on the side.
7. Enjoy this flavorful and healthy meal of baked salmon with dill sauce and roasted asparagus!

Nutrition Value (Per Serving)

Calories: 300 kcal - Carbohydrates: 10g - Protein: 25g - Fat: 15g - Fiber: 5g
- Sugar: 4g - Sodium: 40mg

GRILLED VEGETABLE AND CHICKPEA SALAD

Preparation Time : 15 min

Cooking Time : 15 min

Servings : 4

Ingredients

- 2 cups mixed vegetables (such as bell peppers, zucchini, eggplant, and cherry tomatoes), sliced
- 1 can (15 oz) chickpeas, drained and rinsed
- 2 tablespoons olive oil
- Salt and pepper to taste
- 4 cups mixed greens (such as spinach, arugula, and lettuce)
- 1/4 cup chopped fresh parsley
- 1 lemon, juiced
- 2 tablespoons extra virgin olive oil

Preparation

1. Preheat the grill to medium-high heat.
2. In a bowl, toss the mixed vegetables and chickpeas with olive oil, salt, and pepper until evenly coated.
3. Grill the vegetables and chickpeas for 8-10 minutes, turning occasionally, until charred and tender.
4. In a large salad bowl, combine the grilled vegetables and chickpeas with mixed greens and chopped fresh parsley.
5. In a small bowl, whisk together lemon juice and extra virgin olive oil to make the vinaigrette.
6. Drizzle the lemon vinaigrette over the salad and toss gently to coat.
7. Serve immediately and enjoy this refreshing and nutritious grilled vegetable and chickpea salad!

Nutrition Value (Per Serving)

Calories: 250 kcal- Carbohydrates: 25g - Protein: 8g - Fat: 15g - Fiber: 6g
- Sugar: 4g - Sodium: 30mg

HONEY MUSTARD GLAZED PORK CHOPS WITH ROASTED BRUSSELS SPROUTS

Preparation Time : 15 min

Cooking Time : 25 min

Servings : 2

Ingredients

- 2 pork chops
- 1 tablespoon honey
- 1 tablespoon Dijon mustard
- 1 tablespoon olive oil
- Salt and pepper to taste
- 2 cups Brussels sprouts, trimmed and halved
- 1 tablespoon balsamic vinegar
- 1 tablespoon olive oil
- Salt and pepper to taste

Preparation

1. Preheat the oven to 400°F (200°C).
2. In a small bowl, whisk together honey, Dijon mustard, and olive oil to make the glaze for the pork chops.
3. Sprinkle salt and pepper over both sides of the pork chops.
4. Brush the honey mustard glaze over the pork chops.
5. Arrange the pork chops on a parchment paper-lined baking pan.
6. In a separate bowl, toss Brussels sprouts with balsamic vinegar, olive oil, salt, and pepper.
7. Arrange the Brussels sprouts on the same baking sheet around the pork chops.
8. Bake in the preheated oven for 20-25 minutes, or until the pork chops are cooked through and the Brussels sprouts are tender and caramelized.
9. Serve the honey mustard glazed pork chops with roasted Brussels sprouts.
10. Enjoy this delicious and satisfying meal!

Nutrition Value (Per Serving)

Calories: 350 kcal - Carbohydrates: 20g - Protein: 25g - Fat: 20g - Fiber: 8g - Sugar: 8g - Sodium: 40mg

LEMON GARLIC HERB TILAPIA WITH ROASTED POTATOES AND GREEN BEANS

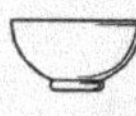 **Preparation Time : 15 min**

 **Cooking Time : 25 min**

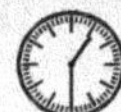 **Servings : 2**

Ingredients

- 2 tilapia fillets
- 2 tablespoons olive oil
- 2 cloves garlic, minced
- 1 tablespoon lemon juice
- 1 teaspoon dried mixed herbs (such as thyme, rosemary, and oregano)
- Salt and pepper to taste
- 2 cups baby potatoes, halved
- 1 cup green beans, trimmed
- Fresh parsley for garnish (optional)

Preparation

1. Preheat the oven to 400°F (200°C).
2. In a small bowl, mix together olive oil, minced garlic, lemon juice, dried mixed herbs, salt, and pepper.
3. Place the tilapia fillets in a baking dish. Brush the garlic herb mixture over the tilapia.
4. On a separate baking sheet, spread out the halved baby potatoes and trimmed green beans. Add a drizzle of olive oil and season with pepper and salt.
5. When the oven is heated, put both baking dishes in.
6. Bake the tilapia for 15-20 minutes, or until cooked through and flakes easily with a fork.
7. Bake the potatoes and green beans for 20-25 minutes, or until tender and golden.
8. Once cooked, remove from the oven and garnish with fresh parsley if desired.
9. Serve the lemon garlic herb tilapia with roasted potatoes and green beans.
10. Enjoy this flavorful and nutritious meal

Nutrition Value (Per Serving)

Calories: 350 kcal - Carbohydrates: 30g - Protein: 25g - Fat: 15g - Fiber: 6g - Sugar: 3g - Sodium: 40mg

CHICKEN AND VEGETABLE SKEWERS WITH GREEK YOGURT TZATZIKI SAUCE

Preparation Time : 20 min

Cooking Time : 15 min

Servings : 2

Ingredients

- 2 boneless, skinless chicken breasts, cut into cubes
- 1 bell pepper, cut into chunks
- 1 zucchini, sliced
- 1 red onion, cut into chunks
- 8 cherry tomatoes
- 2 tablespoons olive oil
- 1 tablespoon lemon juice
- 1 teaspoon dried oregano
- Salt and pepper to taste
- Soak wooden skewers in water for 30 minutes.
- 1/2 cup Greek yogurt
- 1/4 cup grated cucumber
- 1 clove garlic, minced
- 1 tablespoon lemon juice
- 1 tablespoon chopped fresh dill
- Salt and pepper to taste

Preparation

1. Preheat the grill to medium-high heat.
2. In a bowl, mix together olive oil, lemon juice, dried oregano, salt, and pepper. Toss the chicken cubes in the basin until uniformly coated.
3. Thread marinated chicken cubes, bell pepper chunks, zucchini slices, red onion chunks, and cherry tomatoes onto the soaked wooden skewers.
4. Grill the skewers for 10-15 minutes, turning occasionally, until the chicken is cooked through and the vegetables are charred and tender.
5. While the skewers are grilling, prepare the tzatziki sauce. In a small bowl, mix together Greek yogurt, grated cucumber, minced garlic, lemon juice, chopped fresh dill, salt, and pepper.
6. Serve the chicken and vegetable skewers with Greek yogurt tzatziki sauce on the side.
7. Enjoy this delicious and healthy dish!

Nutrition Value (Per Serving)

Calories: 300 kcal - Carbohydrates: 15g - Protein: 25g - Fat: 15g - Fiber: 4g - Sugar: 7g - Sodium: 40mg

RATATOUILLE

☐ **Preparation Time : 20 min**

✗ **Cooking Time : 30 min**

🕐 **Servings : 4**

Ingredients

- 1 eggplant, diced
- 2 zucchinis, diced
- 1 red bell pepper, diced
- 1 yellow bell pepper, diced
- 2 tomatoes, diced
- 1 onion, diced
- 2 cloves garlic, minced
- 2 tablespoons olive oil
- 1 teaspoon dried thyme
- 1 teaspoon dried oregano
- Salt and pepper to taste
- Fresh basil leaves for garnish (optional)

Preparation

1. In a large skillet, heat olive oil over medium heat.
2. Add diced onion and minced garlic. Cook until softened, about 5 minutes.
3. Add diced eggplant, zucchinis, bell peppers, and tomatoes to the skillet. Cook the vegetables for 15-20 minutes, stirring regularly, until soft.
4. Season with dried thyme, dried oregano, salt, and pepper. Stir to combine.
5. Once cooked, remove from heat and transfer the ratatouille to a serving dish.
6. Garnish with fresh basil leaves if desired.
7. Serve hot or at room temperature.
8. Enjoy this classic French dish of ratatouille with eggplant, zucchini, bell peppers, and tomatoes!

Nutrition Value (Per Serving)

Calories: 150 kcal - Carbohydrates: 15g - Protein: 3g - Fat: 10g - Fiber: 5g
- Sugar: 8g - Sodium: 40mg

MEDITERRANEAN STUFFED EGGPLANT

🥣 **Preparation Time : 20 min**

🍴 **Cooking Time : 40 min**

🕐 **Servings : 2**

Ingredients

- 1 large eggplant
- 1/2 cup cooked quinoa
- 1/4 cup crumbled feta cheese
- 2 tablespoons chopped fresh parsley
- 2 tablespoons chopped fresh mint
- 2 tablespoons chopped sun-dried tomatoes
- 1 tablespoon lemon juice
- 2 cloves garlic, minced
- 1 tablespoon olive oil
- Salt and pepper to taste

Preparation

1. Preheat the oven to 375°F (190°C).
2. Slice the eggplant in half lengthwise and scoop out the flesh, leaving about a 1/2-inch border around the edges. Cut the scooped-out flesh into small pieces.
3. In a skillet, heat olive oil over medium heat. Add minced garlic and chopped eggplant flesh. Cook for 5-7 minutes until softened.
4. In a bowl, combine cooked quinoa, crumbled feta cheese, chopped fresh parsley, chopped fresh mint, chopped sun-dried tomatoes, lemon juice, and the cooked eggplant mixture. Season with salt and pepper to taste.
5. Stuff the hollowed-out eggplant halves with the quinoa mixture.
6. Arrange the filled eggplant halves onto a parchment paper-lined baking sheet.
7. Bake in the preheated oven for 30-35 minutes, or until the eggplant is tender and the filling is heated through.
8. Serve hot and enjoy this flavorful and nutritious Mediterranean stuffed eggplant!

Nutrition Value (Per Serving)

Calories: 250 kcal - Carbohydrates: 30g - Protein: 8g - Fat: 12g - Fiber: 10g - Sugar: 6g - Sodium: 40mg

BEEF AND BROCCOLI STIR-FRY

Preparation Time : 15 min

Cooking Time : 15 min

Servings : 2

Ingredients

- 1/2 lb. beef sirloin, thinly sliced
- 2 cups broccoli florets
- 1 red bell pepper, sliced
- 2 cloves garlic, minced
- 2 tablespoons soy sauce (low-sodium)
- 1 tablespoon oyster sauce
- 1 tablespoon sesame oil
- 1 tablespoon cornstarch
- 1/4 cup water
- 1 tablespoon olive oil
- Sesame seeds for garnish (optional)

Preparation

1. In a bowl, mix together soy sauce, oyster sauce, sesame oil, cornstarch, and water to make the sauce.
2. In a large skillet or wok, heat the olive oil over medium-high heat. Add minced garlic and sliced beef. Stir-fry for 2-3 minutes until browned.
3. Add broccoli florets and sliced red bell pepper to the skillet. Stir-fry the vegetables for an additional three to four minutes, or until they are crisp-tender.
4. Pour the sauce over the beef and vegetables in the skillet. Stir to coat evenly. Cook for 2-3 minutes until the sauce thickens.
5. Remove from heat and garnish with sesame seeds if desired.
6. Serve hot and enjoy this delicious beef and broccoli stir-fry!

Nutrition Value (Per Serving)

Calories: 300 kcal - Carbohydrates: 15g - Protein: 25g - Fat: 15g - Fiber: 5g - Sugar: 6g - Sodium: 40mg

Dessert Recipes

CHOCOLATE CHIA PUDDING

Preparation Time : 5 min

Chilling Time : 2 hours

Servings : 2

Ingredients

- 1/4 cup chia seeds
- 1 cup unsweetened almond milk
- 2 tablespoons cocoa powder
- 1 tablespoon maple syrup (optional)
- 1/2 teaspoon vanilla extract
- Fresh berries for garnish (optional)

Preparation

1. In a bowl, mix together chia seeds, unsweetened almond milk, cocoa powder, maple syrup (if using), and vanilla extract until well combined.
2. Cover the bowl and chill for at least 2 hours, preferably overnight, until the chia pudding thickens.
3. Stir the chia pudding before serving to evenly distribute the ingredients.
4. Divide the chocolate chia pudding into serving glasses or bowls.
5. Garnish with fresh berries if desired.
6. Serve chilled and enjoy this indulgent and nutritious chocolate chia pudding!

Nutrition Value (Per Serving)

Calories: 150 kcal- Carbohydrates: 15g - Protein: 5g- Fat: 9g- Fiber: 8g - Sugar: 2g - Sodium: 40mg

CHOCOLATE BROWNIES

◡ **Preparation Time : 10 min**

✕ **Baking Time : 25 min**

◷ **Servings : 9**

Ingredients

- 1/2 cup almond flour
- 1/4 cup cocoa powder
- 1/4 cup maple syrup
- 1/4 cup coconut oil, melted
- 2 tablespoons unsweetened almond milk
- 1 teaspoon vanilla extract
- 1/4 teaspoon baking powder
- Pinch of salt
- Chopped nuts for garnish (optional)

Preparation

1. Preheat the oven to 350°F (175°C). Grease a square baking pan and line it with parchment paper.
2. In a bowl, whisk together almond flour, cocoa powder, maple syrup, melted coconut oil, unsweetened almond milk, vanilla extract, baking powder, and a pinch of salt until smooth.
3. Pour the batter into the prepared baking pan and spread it evenly.
4. Sprinkle chopped nuts on top if desired.
5. Bake in the preheated oven for 20-25 minutes, or until the brownies are set and a toothpick inserted into the center comes out clean.
6. Remove from the oven and let the brownies cool completely in the pan before slicing.
7. Once cooled, slice into squares and serve.
8. Enjoy these decadent and fudgy chocolate brownies guilt-free!

Nutrition Value (Per Serving)

Calories: 150 kcal - Carbohydrates: 10g - Protein: 2g - Fat: 12g - Fiber: 3g - Sugar: 6g - Sodium: 40mg

PEANUT BUTTER BANANA PANCAKES

Preparation Time : 10 min

Cooking Time : 10 min

Servings : 2

Ingredients

- 1 ripe banana
- 2 eggs
- 2 tablespoons peanut butter
- 1/4 teaspoon cinnamon
- 1/4 teaspoon vanilla extract
- Coconut oil for cooking
- Sliced bananas and maple syrup for serving (optional)

Preparation

1. In a bowl, mash the ripe banana with a fork until smooth.
2. Add eggs, peanut butter, cinnamon, and vanilla extract to the mashed banana. Whisk until well combined.
3. Heat coconut oil in a skillet over medium heat.
4. Pour pancake batter onto the skillet to form small pancakes.
5. Cook for 2-3 minutes on each side, until golden brown and cooked through.
6. Remove from the skillet and repeat with the remaining batter.
7. Serve the peanut butter banana pancakes with sliced bananas and maple syrup if desired.
8. Enjoy these fluffy and flavorful pancakes for a delicious breakfast or brunch!

Nutrition Value (Per Serving)

Calories: 250 kcal - Carbohydrates: 20g - Protein: 10g - Fat: 15g - Fiber: 3g - Sugar: 8g - Sodium: 40mg

FERRERO ROCHER

🥣 **Preparation Time : 20 min**

✖ **Chilling Time : 1 hour**

🕐 **Servings : 12**

Ingredients

- 1/2 cup hazelnuts
- 12 whole roasted hazelnuts
- 1/4 cup cocoa powder
- 1/4 cup powdered sugar
- 1/4 cup coconut oil, melted
- 1/2 teaspoon vanilla extract
- Pinch of salt

Preparation

1. Preheat the oven to 350°F (175°C).
2. Spread hazelnuts on a baking sheet and roast for 10-12 minutes, until fragrant.
3. Remove from the oven and let the hazelnuts cool slightly. Rub them with a kitchen towel to remove the skins.
4. In a food processor, blend roasted hazelnuts until finely ground.
5. Add cocoa powder, powdered sugar, melted coconut oil, vanilla extract, and a pinch of salt to the ground hazelnuts. Blend until a smooth paste forms.
6. Take small portions of the hazelnut mixture and wrap around each roasted hazelnut to form balls.
7. Place the balls on a parchment-lined tray and refrigerate for at least 1 hour to set.
8. Once set, serve and enjoy these homemade Ferrero Rocher chocolates!

Nutrition Value (Per Serving)

Calories: 120 kcal - Carbohydrates: 5g - Protein: 2g- Fat: 10g - Fiber: 2g
- Sugar: 2g - Sodium: 30mg

PALEO MOCHA FRAPPUCCINO

Preparation Time : 5 min

Cooking Time : 0 min

Servings : 1

Ingredients

- 1 cup brewed coffee, chilled
- 1/2 cup coconut milk
- 1 tablespoon cocoa powder
- 1 tablespoon maple syrup (optional)
- 1/2 teaspoon vanilla extract
- Ice cubes
- Cocoa powder for garnish (optional)

Preparation

1. In a blender, combine chilled brewed coffee, coconut milk, cocoa powder, maple syrup (if using), vanilla extract, and a handful of ice cubes.
2. Blend until smooth and creamy.
3. Pour the mocha Frappuccino into a glass.
4. Garnish with a sprinkle of cocoa powder if desired.
5. Serve immediately and enjoy this refreshing paleo-friendly mocha Frappuccino!

Nutrition Value (Per Serving)

Calories: 100 kcal - Carbohydrates: 7g - Protein: 1g - Fat: 8g - Fiber: 1g
- Sugar: 4g - Sodium: 40mg

ALMOND BANANA TART

Preparation Time : 15 min

Cooking Time : 20 min

Servings : 6

Ingredients

- 1 cup almond flour
- 1/4 cup coconut oil, melted
- 2 tablespoons maple syrup
- 1/4 teaspoon almond extract
- 2 ripe bananas, sliced
- 1 tablespoon lemon juice
- Sliced almonds for garnish (optional)

Preparation

1. Preheat the oven to 350°F (175°C). Grease a tart pan.
2. In a bowl, combine almond flour, melted coconut oil, maple syrup, and almond extract. Mix until a dough forms.
3. Press the dough into the bottom and up the sides of the tart pan to form a crust.
4. Bake the crust in the preheated oven for 10-12 minutes, until lightly golden. Let it cool completely.
5. In a bowl, toss sliced bananas with lemon juice to prevent browning.
6. Arrange the sliced bananas on top of the cooled almond crust.
7. Refrigerate the almond banana tart for at least 1 hour to set.
8. Garnish with sliced almonds before serving if desired.
9. Slice and serve this delicious almond banana tart!

Nutrition Value (Per Serving)

Calories: 200 kcal - Carbohydrates: 15g - Protein: 3g - Fat: 15g - Fiber: 3g - Sugar: 8g - Sodium: 40mg

MANGO CRUMBLE

Preparation Time : 15 min

Cooking Time : 25 min

Servings : 4

Ingredients

- 2 ripe mangoes, peeled and diced
- 1 tablespoon lemon juice
- 1/2 cup almond flour
- 2 tablespoons coconut oil, melted
- 2 tablespoons maple syrup
- 1/4 teaspoon ground cinnamon
- Pinch of salt

Preparation

1. Preheat the oven to 375°F (190°C). Grease a baking dish.
2. In a bowl, toss diced mangoes with lemon juice. Transfer to the prepared baking dish.
3. In another bowl, combine almond flour, melted coconut oil, maple syrup, ground cinnamon, and a pinch of salt. Mix until crumbly.
4. Sprinkle the almond crumble mixture over the diced mangoes in the baking dish.
5. Bake in the preheated oven for 20-25 minutes, until the crumble topping is golden brown and the mangoes are bubbling.
6. Remove from the oven and allow it cool slightly.
7. Serve warm or at room temperature.
8. Enjoy this delightful mango crumble as a dessert or snack!

Nutrition Value (Per Serving)

Calories: 180 kcal - Carbohydrates: 20g Protein: 2g - Fat: 12g - Fiber: 3g - Sugar: 15g - Sodium: 40mg

BANANA ICE CREAM

Preparation Time : 5 min

Freezing Time : 4 hours

Servings : 2

Ingredients

- 2 ripe bananas, sliced and frozen
- 2 tablespoons unsweetened almond milk
- 1 teaspoon vanilla extract
- Optional toppings: sliced bananas, chopped nuts, cocoa powder

Preparation

1. Put the frozen banana slices in a food processor or blender.
2. Add unsweetened almond milk and vanilla extract.
3. Blend until smooth and creamy, scraping down the sides of the blender or food processor as needed.
4. Add extra almond milk, one tablespoon at a time, if the mixture is too thick, until the right consistency is achieved.
5. Transfer the banana ice cream to a container and freeze for at least 4 hours, or until firm.
6. Before serving, let the banana ice cream sit at room temperature for a few minutes to soften slightly.
7. Scoop into bowls and garnish with your favorite toppings if desired.
8. Enjoy this creamy and delicious banana ice cream guilt-free!

Nutrition Value (Per Serving)

Calories: 100 kcal - Carbohydrates: 25g - Protein: 1g - Fat: 0.5g - Fiber: 3g - Sugar: 14g - Sodium: 0mg

BAKED APPLES

Preparation Time : 10 min

Baking Time : 30 min

Servings : 2

Ingredients

- 2 apples (such as Granny Smith or Honeycrisp)
- 2 tablespoons chopped walnuts
- 1 tablespoon maple syrup
- 1/2 teaspoon ground cinnamon
- 1/4 teaspoon nutmeg
- Pinch of salt
- Fresh mint leaves for garnish (optional)

Preparation

1. Preheat the oven to 375°F (190°C).
2. Keep the bottoms of the apples whole while you wash and core them.
3. In a small bowl, mix together chopped walnuts, maple syrup, ground cinnamon, nutmeg, and a pinch of salt.
4. Stuff each apple with the walnut mixture.
5. Arrange the filled apples into a baking tray.
6. Bake in the preheated oven for 25-30 minutes, until the apples are tender and the filling is golden brown.
7. Remove from the oven and let the baked apples cool slightly.
8. If desired, garnish with fresh mint leaves.
9. Serve warm and enjoy these delicious baked apples as a healthy dessert!

Nutrition Value (Per Serving)

Calories: 150 kcal - Carbohydrates: 25g - Protein: 2g - Fat: 6g - Fiber: 5g - Sugar: 18g - Sodium: 0mg

CHOCOLATE AVOCADO MOUSSE WITH FRESH BERRIES

⬤ **Preparation Time : 10 min**

✖ **Chilling Time : 1 hour**

🕐 **Servings : 2**

Ingredients

- 1 ripe avocado
- 2 tablespoons cocoa powder
- 2 tablespoons maple syrup
- 1/2 teaspoon vanilla extract
- Fresh berries for serving (such as strawberries, raspberries, or blueberries)
- Mint leaves for garnish (optional)

Preparation

1. Scoop the flesh of the ripe avocado into a blender or food processor.
2. Add cocoa powder, maple syrup, and vanilla extract.
3. Blend until smooth and creamy, scraping down the sides of the blender or food processor as needed.
4. Transfer the chocolate avocado mousse to serving glasses or bowls.
5. Cover and refrigerate for at least 1 hour to chill.
6. Before serving, top with fresh berries and garnish with mint leaves if desired.
7. Enjoy this rich and indulgent chocolate avocado mousse as a guilt-free dessert!

Nutrition Value (Per Serving)

Calories: 200 kcal - Carbohydrates: 20g - Protein: 3g - Fat: 14g - Fiber: 7g - Sugar: 10g - Sodium: 5mg

LEMON SORBET WITH FRESH MINT LEAVES

🥣 **Preparation Time : 10 min**

✂️ **Chilling Time : 4 hours**

🕐 **Servings : 4**

Ingredients

- 1 cup water
- 1/2 cup freshly squeezed lemon juice
- 1/2 cup maple syrup
- Zest of 1 lemon
- Fresh mint leaves for garnish (optional)

Preparation

1. In a bowl, mix together water, freshly squeezed lemon juice, maple syrup, and lemon zest until well combined.
2. Pour the mixture into a shallow dish or ice cube tray.
3. Cover and freeze for about 2 hours, or until partially frozen.
4. Remove from the freezer and break up the mixture with a fork to break up any ice crystals.
5. Return the mixture to the freezer and freeze for another 2 hours, or until completely frozen.
6. Before serving, let the sorbet sit at room temperature for a few minutes to soften slightly.
7. Scoop the lemon sorbet into serving bowls or glasses.
8. If desired, garnish with fresh mint leaves.
9. Serve immediately and enjoy this refreshing lemon sorbet!

Nutrition Value (Per Serving)

Calories: 120 kcal - Carbohydrates: 30g - Protein: 0g - Fat: 0g - Fiber: 1g - Sugar: 25g - Sodium: 0mg

COCONUT MILK RICE PUDDING

<table>
<tr><td>Preparation Time : 5 min</td></tr>
<tr><td>Cooking Time : 30 min</td></tr>
<tr><td>Servings : 4</td></tr>
</table>

Ingredients

- 1/2 cup white rice
- 1 can (13.5 oz) coconut milk
- 2 cups water
- 1/4 cup maple syrup
- 1 teaspoon vanilla extract
- 1/4 teaspoon ground cinnamon
- Pinch of salt
- Shredded coconut for garnish (optional)

Preparation

1. In a saucepan, combine white rice, coconut milk, water, maple syrup, vanilla extract, ground cinnamon, and a pinch of salt.
2. On medium heat, bring the mixture to a boil.
3. Reduce the heat to low and simmer, stirring occasionally, for about 25-30 minutes, or until the rice is cooked and the mixture has thickened.
4. Take the rice pudding from the flame and allow it to cool slightly.
5. Transfer the rice pudding to serving bowls or glasses.
6. Refrigerate for at least two hours, or until cool.
7. Before serving, garnish with shredded coconut if desired.
8. Enjoy this creamy and delicious coconut milk rice pudding as a comforting dessert or snack!

Nutrition Value (Per Serving)

Calories: 250 kcal - Carbohydrates: 30g - Protein: 3g - Fat: 13g - Fiber: 1g
- Sugar: 10g - Sodium: 30mg

BAKED PEACHES

⬤ **Preparation Time : 10 min**

✖ **Baking Time : 20 min**

🕐 **Servings : 2**

Ingredients

- 2 ripe peaches, halved and pitted
- 2 tablespoons honey
- 1/4 cup almond flour
- 2 tablespoons rolled oats
- 2 tablespoons chopped almonds
- 1 tablespoon coconut oil, melted
- 1/4 teaspoon ground cinnamon
- Pinch of salt

Preparation

1. Preheat the oven to 375°F (190°C). Grease a baking dish.
2. Place peach halves, cut side up, in the prepared baking dish.
3. Drizzle honey over the peach halves.
4. In a bowl, combine almond flour, rolled oats, chopped almonds, melted coconut oil, ground cinnamon, and a pinch of salt. Mix until crumbly.
5. Sprinkle the almond crumble mixture over the honey-drizzled peach halves.
6. Bake in the preheated oven for 15-20 minutes, or until the peaches are tender and the crumble topping is golden brown.
7. Remove from the oven and let the baked peaches cool slightly.
8. Serve warm and enjoy these delicious baked peaches with honey and almond crumble topping!

Nutrition Value (Per Serving)

Calories: 200 kcal - Carbohydrates: 25g - Protein: 3g - Fat: 11g - Fiber: 4g - Sugar: 19g - Sodium: 20mg

MANGO COCONUT CHIA POPSICLES

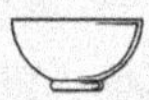 **Preparation Time : 10 min**

 **Freezing Time : 4 hours**

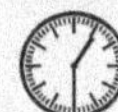 **Servings : 6**

Ingredients

- 2 ripe mangoes, peeled and diced
- 1 can (13.5 oz) coconut milk
- 1/4 cup chia seeds
- 2 tablespoons maple syrup
- 1 teaspoon vanilla extract
- Popsicle molds
- Popsicle sticks

Preparation

1. In a blender, puree diced mangoes until smooth.
2. In a bowl, mix together pureed mangoes, coconut milk, chia seeds, maple syrup, and vanilla extract until well combined.
3. Pour the mango coconut chia mixture into popsicle molds.
4. Insert popsicle sticks into each mold.
5. Freeze for at least 4 hours, or until the popsicles are completely frozen.
6. Once frozen, remove the popsicles from the molds by running them under warm water for a few seconds.
7. Serve immediately and enjoy these refreshing mango coconut chia popsicles on a hot day!

Nutrition Value (Per Serving)

Calories: 150 kcal - Carbohydrates: 20g - Protein: 2g - Fat: 8g - Fiber: 4g
- Sugar: 14g - Sodium: 20mg

PUMPKIN SPICE ENERGY BITES

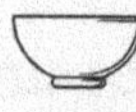 **Preparation Time : 15 min**

 **Chilling Time : 30 min**

 **Servings : 12**

Ingredients

- 1 cup rolled oats
- 1/2 cup pumpkin puree
- 1/4 cup almond butter
- 1/4 cup chopped dates
- 2 tablespoons maple syrup
- 1 teaspoon pumpkin pie spice
- 1/4 cup shredded coconut (optional)

Preparation

1. In a large bowl, combine rolled oats, pumpkin puree, almond butter, chopped dates, maple syrup, and pumpkin pie spice.
2. Mix until well combined.
3. If the mixture is too wet, add more rolled oats.
4. If it's too dry, add a bit more almond butter or maple syrup.
5. Using your hands, roll the mixture into small balls, about 1 inch in diameter.
6. If desired, roll the energy bites in shredded coconut to coat.
7. Place the energy bites on a baking sheet lined with parchment paper.
8. Chill in the refrigerator for at least 30 minutes to firm up.
9. Once chilled, store the pumpkin spice energy bites in an airtight container in the refrigerator for up to one week.
10. Enjoy these delicious and nutritious energy bites as a quick snack or pre-workout boost!

Nutrition Value (Per Serving)

Calories: 80 kcal - Carbohydrates: 10g - Protein: 2g - Fat: 4g - Fiber: 2g - Sugar: 4g - Sodium: 0mg

GREEK YOGURT POPSICLES WITH MANGO AND PINEAPPLE

Preparation Time : 10 min

Freezing Time : 4 hours

Servings : 6

Ingredients

- 1 cup Greek yogurt
- 1/2 cup diced mango
- 1/2 cup diced pineapple
- 2 tablespoons honey or maple syrup

Preparation

1. In a bowl, mix together Greek yogurt and honey or maple syrup until smooth.
2. Divide the diced mango and pineapple among popsicle molds.
3. Pour the Greek yogurt mixture over the fruit in the molds, filling them to the top.
4. Insert popsicle sticks into each mold.
5. Freeze for at least 4 hours, or until the popsicles are completely frozen.
6. Once frozen, remove the popsicles from the molds by running them under warm water for a few seconds.
7. Serve immediately and enjoy these refreshing Greek yogurt popsicles with mango and pineapple!

Nutrition Value (Per Serving)

Calories: 70 kcal - Carbohydrates: 12g - Protein: 4g - Fat: 1g - Fiber: 1g - Sugar: 10g - Sodium: 20mg

ROASTED CHICKPEAS

Preparation Time : 5 min

Cooking Time : 30 min

Servings : 4

Ingredients

- 1 can (15 oz) chickpeas, drained and rinsed
- 1 tablespoon olive oil
- 1 teaspoon paprika
- 1/2 teaspoon garlic powder
- Salt to taste

Preparation

1. Preheat the oven to 400°F (200°C). Line a baking sheet with parchment paper.
2. Pat the chickpeas dry with a clean kitchen towel or paper towels to remove excess moisture.
3. In a bowl, toss the dried chickpeas with olive oil, paprika, garlic powder, and salt until evenly coated.
4. Spread the seasoned chickpeas in a single layer on the prepared baking sheet.
5. Roast in the preheated oven for 25-30 minutes, shaking the pan occasionally, until the chickpeas are golden brown and crispy.
6. Remove from the oven and let the roasted chickpeas cool slightly before serving.
7. Enjoy these crunchy and flavorful roasted chickpeas as a healthy snack or salad topper!

Nutrition Value (Per Serving)

Calories: 120 kcal - Carbohydrates: 15g - Protein: 5g - Fat: 4g - Fiber: 4g - Sugar: 1g- Sodium: 10mg

TRAIL MIX

🥣 **Preparation Time : 5 min**

🍴 **Cooking Time : 0 min**

🕐 **Servings : 4**

Ingredients

- 1/2 cup mixed nuts (such as almonds, cashews, and walnuts)
- 1/4 cup dried fruit (such as raisins, cranberries, or apricots), chopped if large
- 2 tablespoons dark chocolate chips

Preparation

1. In a bowl, mix together mixed nuts, dried fruit, and dark chocolate chips until well combined.
2. Divide the trail mix into individual servings or store in an airtight container for later enjoyment.
3. Enjoy this delicious and nutritious trail mix as a convenient snack on the go!

Nutrition Value (Per Serving)

Calories: 150 kcal- Carbohydrates: 15g - Protein: 4g - Fat: 9g - Fiber: 3g - Sugar: 8g - Sodium: 0mg

HUMMUS WITH CARROT AND CUCUMBER STICKS

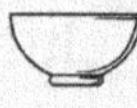 **Preparation Time : 5 min**

 **Cooking Time : 0 min**

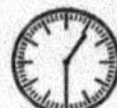 **Servings : 1**

Ingredients

- 2 tablespoons hummus (store-bought or homemade)
- 1 carrot, cut into sticks
- 1 cucumber, cut into sticks

Preparation

1. Place the hummus in a small bowl or serving container.
2. Arrange the carrot and cucumber sticks on a plate or serving tray.
3. Serve the hummus alongside the carrot and cucumber sticks for a delicious and nutritious snack or appetizer.
4. Dip the crunchy vegetables into the creamy hummus for a satisfying combination of flavors and textures!

Nutrition Value (Per Serving)

Calories: 70 kcal - Carbohydrates: 10g - Protein: 3g - Fat: 2g - Fiber: 4g - Sugar: 4g- Sodium: 40mg

WEEK ONE

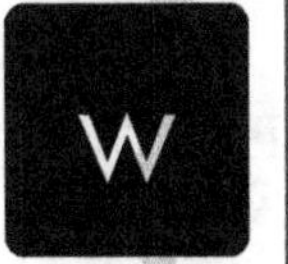

	Breakfast:	Lunch:	Dinner:	Snack:
s	**Banana Bread Oatmeal**	**Chickpea Noodle Soup**	**Black Beans Quesadilla**	**Hummus with Carrot and Cucumber Sticks**
m	**Oat Waffles**	**Zoodle Pad Thai**	**Lemon Herb Chicken with Steamed Broccoli and Brown Rice**	**Trail Mix**
t	**Cinnamon Apple Parfaits**	**Spinach and Pear Salad**	**Turkey Meatballs with Zucchini Noodles**	**Chocolate Chia Pudding**
w	**Breakfast Tostadas**	**Roasted Sweet Potato and Black Bean Nachos**	**Pan-Roasted Mackerel with Vegetables**	**Greek Yogurt Popsicles with Mango and Pineapple**
t	**Mediterranean Baked Sweet Potatoes**	**Vegetable Curry**	**Grilled Vegetable and Chickpea Salad**	**Roasted Chickpeas**
f	**Quinoa Breakfast Bowl with Fresh Berries**	**Vegetable Fried Rice**	**Ratatouille**	**Baked Peaches**
s	**Spinach and Mushroom Omelette with Avocado Slices**	**Pear and Walnut Grain Salad**	**Baked Salmon with Dill Sauce and Roasted Asparagus**	**Banana Ice Cream**

WEEK TWO

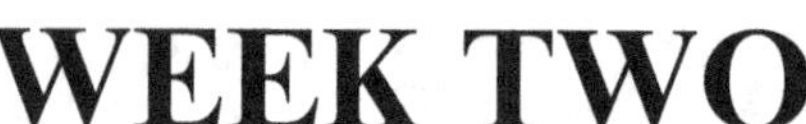

	Breakfast:	Lunch:	Dinner:	Snack:
s	**Overnight Chia Seed Pudding**	**Mediterranean Chickpea Stew**	**Honey Mustard Glazed Pork Chops with Roasted Brussels Sprouts**	**Pumpkin Spice Energy Bites**
m	**Buckwheat Pancakes with Blueberry Compote**	**Vegetable Soup**	**Curry Corn Chowder**	**Coconut Milk Rice Pudding**
t	**Egg Muffins**	**Sweet Corn and Black Bean Tacos**	**Lemon Garlic Herb Tilapia with Roasted Potatoes and Green Beans**	**Mango Coconut Chia Popsicles**
w	**Breakfast Burrito**	**Stuffed Bell Peppers**	**Chicken and Vegetable Skewers with Greek Yogurt Tzatziki Sauce**	**Pumpkin Spice Energy Bites**
t	**Acai Bowl**	**Lentil Soup**	**Mediterranean Stuffed Eggplant**	**Lemon Sorbet with Fresh Mint Leaves**
f	**Turmeric Scrambled Tofu**	**Veggie Sushi Rolls**	**Beef and Broccoli Stir-Fry**	**Almond Banana Tart**
s	**Breakfast Quinoa Porridge with Apple Cinnamon Compote**	**Turkey and Vegetable Stir-Fry with Brown Rice**	**Kale, Smoked Trout, and Avocado Salad**	**Chocolate Avocado Mousse with Fresh Berries**

CONCLUSION

The recipes and meal plans provided in this lupus diet cookbook offer a comprehensive and practical approach to managing lupus symptoms through nutrition.

By focusing on nutrient-dense, whole foods and avoiding potential inflammatory triggers, you can support your body's immune function, reduce inflammation, and promote overall health.

The recipes have been carefully chosen to cater to a variety of tastes and preferences while ensuring that they adhere to the principles of a lupus-friendly diet.

Whether you are new to cooking or experienced in the kitchen, these meals are designed to be easy to prepare and incorporate into your daily routine.

Meal prep tips in the cookbook help you save time and stay on track with your dietary goals. By planning ahead and preparing meals in advance, you can maintain a balanced diet even on your busiest days.

Remember, managing lupus through diet is a personalized journey, and it's essential to listen to your body and work with your healthcare provider to tailor your diet to your unique needs. This cookbook serves as a valuable resource to help you take control of your health and well-being.

I hope these recipes inspire you to explore new flavors, experiment with fresh ingredients, and find joy in the process of nourishing your body. May this cookbook be a supportive companion on your journey towards a healthier and happier life.

WEEKLY MEAL PLANNER

WEEK:

DATE:

MONDAY

TUESDAY

WEDNESDAY

THURSDAY

FRIDAY

SATURDAY

SUNDAY

MOTIVATION FOR THE WEEK

GROCERY LIST FOR THE WEEK

WEEKLY MEAL PLANNER

WEEK:

DATE:

MONDAY

TUESDAY

WEDNESDAY

THURSDAY

FRIDAY

SATURDAY

SUNDAY

MOTIVATION FOR THE WEEK

GROCERY LIST FOR THE WEEK

WEEKLY MEAL PLANNER

WEEK:

DATE:

MONDAY	TUESDAY	WEDNESDAY

THURSDAY	FRIDAY	SATURDAY

SUNDAY

MOTIVATION FOR THE WEEK

GROCERY LIST FOR THE WEEK

WEEKLY MEAL PLANNER

WEEK:

DATE:

MONDAY

TUESDAY

WEDNESDAY

THURSDAY

FRIDAY

SATURDAY

SUNDAY

MOTIVATION FOR THE WEEK

GROCERY LIST FOR THE WEEK

WEEKLY MEAL PLANNER

WEEK:

DATE:

MONDAY

TUESDAY

WEDNESDAY

THURSDAY

FRIDAY

SATURDAY

SUNDAY

MOTIVATION FOR THE WEEK

GROCERY LIST FOR THE WEEK

WEEKLY MEAL PLANNER

WEEK:

DATE:

MONDAY

TUESDAY

WEDNESDAY

THURSDAY

FRIDAY

SATURDAY

SUNDAY

MOTIVATION FOR THE WEEK

GROCERY LIST FOR THE WEEK

WEEKLY MEAL PLANNER

WEEK:

DATE:

MONDAY

TUESDAY

WEDNESDAY

THURSDAY

FRIDAY

SATURDAY

SUNDAY

MOTIVATION FOR THE WEEK

GROCERY LIST FOR THE WEEK

WEEKLY MEAL PLANNER

WEEK:

DATE:

MONDAY

TUESDAY

WEDNESDAY

THURSDAY

FRIDAY

SATURDAY

SUNDAY

MOTIVATION FOR THE WEEK

GROCERY LIST FOR THE WEEK

WEEKLY
MEAL PLANNER

WEEK:

DATE:

MONDAY

TUESDAY

WEDNESDAY

THURSDAY

FRIDAY

SATURDAY

SUNDAY

MOTIVATION FOR THE WEEK

GROCERY LIST FOR THE WEEK

WEEKLY MEAL PLANNER

WEEK: | | DATE: |

MONDAY

TUESDAY

WEDNESDAY

THURSDAY

FRIDAY

SATURDAY

SUNDAY

MOTIVATION FOR THE WEEK

GROCERY LIST FOR THE WEEK